D1621136

Adrian Lussi
Thomas Jaeggi

Dental Erosion

Diagnosis, Risk Assessment, Prevention, Treatment

Adrian Lussi
Thomas Jaeggi

Dental Erosion
Diagnosis, Risk Assessment, Prevention, Treatment

In collaboration with:
Carolina Ganß
Elmar Hellwig

With case reports from:
Carola Imfeld
Nadine Schlueter
Patrick R. Schmidlin
Olivier O. Schicht
Thomas Attin
Anne Grüninger

With a foreword by:
Reinhard Hickel

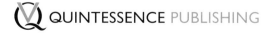

London, Berlin, Chicago, Tokyo, Barcelona, Beijing, Istanbul, Milan,
Moscow, New Delhi, Paris, Prague, São Paulo, Seoul Singapore and Warsaw

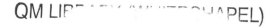
Translated from the original in German titled
Dentale Erosionen: Von der Diagnose zur Therapie
(ISBN: 978-3-938947-08-1).

British Library Cataloguing in Publication Data
Dental erosion : diagnosis, risk assessment, prevention, treatment.
  1. Teeth--Erosion.
  I. Lussi, Adrian. II. Jaeggi, Thomas.
  617.6'3-dc23

ISBN-13: 978-1-85097-218-1

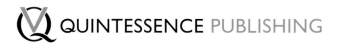

Quintessence Publishing Co. Ltd,
Grafton Road, New Malden, Surrey KT3 3AB,
United Kingdom
www.quintpub.co.uk

Editing: Quintessence Publishing Co. Ltd, London, UK
Layout and Production: Janina Kuhn, Quintessenz Verlags-GmbH, Berlin, Germany
Printed and bound in Germany

Editors and authors

Prof. Dr. med. dent. Adrian Lussi
University of Bern
Department of Preventive,
Restorative and Pediatric Dentistry
Freiburgstrasse 7
CH-3010 Bern, Switzerland

Dr. med. dent. Thomas Jaeggi
University of Bern
Department of Preventive,
Restorative and Pediatric Dentistry
Freiburgstrasse 7
CH-3010 Bern, Switzerland

Prof. Dr. med. dent. Thomas Attin
University of Zurich
Center of Dental Medicine
Clinic of Preventive Dentistry,
Periodontology and Cariology
Plattenstrasse 11
CH-8032 Zurich, Switzerland

Prof. Dr. med. dent. Carolina Ganß
Justus-Liebig University Giessen
Center for Dental, Oral and
Maxillofacial Surgery
Clinic of Conservative and
Preventive Dentistry
Schlangenzahl 14
D-35392 Giessen, Germany

Dr. med. dent. Anne Grüninger
University of Bern
Department of Preventive,
Restorative and Pediatric Dentistry
Freiburgstrasse 7
CH-3010 Bern, Switzerland

Prof. Dr. med. dent. Elmar Hellwig
University Medical Center Freiburg
Clinic for Dental, Oral and
Maxillofacial Surgery
Department of Operative Dentistry
and Periodontology
Hugstetter Straße 55
D-79095 Freiburg, Germany

Dr. med. dent. Carola Imfeld
University of Zurich
Center of Dental Medicine
Clinic of Preventive Dentistry,
Periodontology and Cariology
Plattenstrasse 11
CH-8032 Zurich, Switzerland

Dr. med. dent. Olivier O. Schicht
University of Zurich
Center of Dental Medicine
Clinic of Preventive Dentistry,
Periodontology and Cariology
Plattenstrasse 11
CH-8032 Zurich, Switzerland

Dr. med. dent. Nadine Schlueter
Justus-Liebig University Giessen
Center for Dental, Oral and
Maxillofacial Surgery
Clinic of Conservative and
Preventive Dentistry
Schlangenzahl 14
D-35392 Giessen, Germany

PD Dr. med. dent. Patrick R.
Schmidlin
University of Zurich
Center of Dental Medicine
Clinic of Preventive Dentistry,
Periodontology and Cariology
Plattenstrasse 11
CH-8032 Zurich, Switzerland

Content

Foreword

In the last several decades, there has been a remarkable caries decline in developed countries. This is mainly due to improved oral hygiene and fluorides. However, in the last 25 years in particular, in groups with a higher socio-economic level, health awareness has increased and diet has changed. More and more people are consuming more acidic drinks and juices, and eating fruits or salads with vinegar dressing. These behavior changes and additional factors cause increasing loss of hard tooth tissues by erosion. One problem is that not only the patients but also many dentists do not have sufficient knowledge about this topic and how to prevent and treat this disease.

This book captures the prevalence and multifactorial reasons for erosive tooth substance loss, including the diagnosis, severity index and incidence, progression, and risk factors. Prevention of erosion and therapy adjusted to risk and age, including deciduous teeth, are also covered. This book is illustrated with excellent clinical pictures and step-by-step instructions for the daily practice.

The task of bringing together the current knowledge and understanding of erosion requires exceptional authors with wide-ranging expertise, and an acknowledged and formidable reputation in the field of erosion. Adrian Lussi fits this profile perfectly and he is to be congratulated on having conceived, planned, and edited this book.

The book can be recommended to all practitioners, students, and teachers as a valuable guide for diagnosis, treatment, and prevention of erosion. All those who read and digest the contents of this book will be enlightened and encouraged to widen the scope of their clinical practice and to treat this disease more efficiently with the aim of serving the needs and expectations of patients to the best possible advantage.

Prof. Dr. Reinhard Hickel, Munich

Chapter 1

Introduction

Adrian Lussi and Thomas Jaeggi

The relevance of dental erosion – tooth demineralization without the involvement of bacteria – has increased substantially over recent years. This fact is supported not only by daily observation in dental practice, but also by the large number of academic publications on the subject. In the 1970s, fewer than five publications per year addressed dental erosion, whereas this had doubled to approximately 10 a year in the 1980s. In the late 2000s, there were more than 100 publications on the topic every year. This striking number reflects several factors, including the declining occurrence of caries in recent decades, which has allowed erosion to gain prominence, and altered dietary habits, which have had a marked effect. The consumption of soft drinks has tripled since the late 1980s. Additionally, the manner of consumption has changed, particularly by children and young adults (sipping, sucking on bottles, and through teeth). The increasing occurrence of erosion can be considered a direct consequence of those factors.

The pH of foods and beverages is also of importance; however, it would be wrong to attribute the etiology of erosions to one single factor, where it is clearly a multifaceted process. This book discusses all these aspects with an audience of both students and practitioners in mind. The checklist printed on the next page presents a tool for a systematic approach in examination for dental erosion and its prevention. One chapter collecting contributions by researchers in various university clinics on therapeutic measures shows the full breadth of options and resources currently available for the treatment of dental erosion.

Checklist for dental erosions

Diagnosis   BEWE (basic erosive wear examination)

Etiology

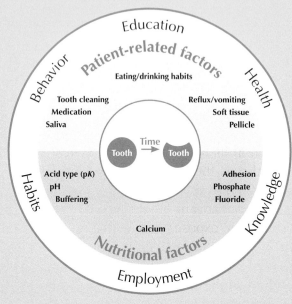

Risk assessment
- Dietary habits
- Frequency and amount of consumption
- Sports and occupational exposure
- Salivary flow rate
- Gastroesophageal reflux
- Bulimia and anorexia

Preventive measures
- Calcium content in foods and beverages
- Products containing (stannous) fluoride
- Changing traumatic tooth-cleaning habits
- Gastroenterological treatment
- Psychological treatment

Treatment
- Protection with bonding systems
- Resin composite
- Ceramic

Follow-up

Chapter 2

Diagnosis of erosion

Adrian Lussi, Carolina Ganß, and Thomas Jaeggi

Summary

Dental erosion in its first stages is difficult to diagnose as the degradation of the enamel surface is usually a gradual process. Only in an advanced stage will concavities and/or exposure of dentin occur, making the lesions clinically clearly visible. The patient will not notice the lesions until teeth turn yellow or begin to shorten through loss of enamel, or when hypersensitivity starts to occur. As a result, it is particularly important for the clinician to be aware of this issue, to be trained in recognizing erosive lesions at an early stage, and to be familiar with preventive measures.

Dental erosion has to be distinguished from other enamel and dentin defects in differential diagnosis. Erosion may occur simultaneously with caries lesions, but never on the same tooth surface at the same time. Erosion is also to be distinguished from mechanically induced defects such as abrasion and attrition, although these conditions often overlap.

In this chapter, the clinical appearance and differential diagnosis of erosion will be discussed. Furthermore, a method for an efficient screening for erosive defects is presented: the basic erosive wear examination (BEWE).[1]

Clinical appearance

The clinical appearance of erosion varies depending on location and changes during the erosive process. Because of structural differences in tooth surfaces, it is difficult to assess the severity of the lesions. For example, erosion near the neck of the tooth or near cavities leads to accelerated exposure of dentin because of the thinness of enamel in those areas. The lesion can appear more pronounced, although in reality no more material may have been lost than in areas where dentin is not yet exposed. This is relevant pathophysiologically, as it is important to know how much tooth substance has been lost. The success rate of preventive measures can only be monitored if the loss of material can be determined initially. By periodically monitoring the erosive defects, the success rate of preventive and/or restorative measures can be longitudinally evaluated. The clinical index developed by Bartlett, Ganß, and Lussi[1] takes these considerations into account and will be described in more detail at a later stage in this chapter. Another method of monitoring the process is to compare photographic images or casts produced periodically.

In contrast to monitoring the loss of the entire tooth substance, it is also clinically important to determine whether dentin is exposed. On the one hand, dentin exposal leads to additional problems for the patient because of hypersensitivity. On the other hand, hypersensitivity can provide valuable information for the clinician with respect to the lesion's status. Disappearing clinical symptoms can indicate success of preventive measures. In addition, discoloration of dentin indicates suspension of substance loss, which can serve as a means of controlling the efficacy of measures taken. However, if hypersensitivity persists and the tooth areas show no discoloration, a continuation of the erosive process is likely.

Initial stages of dental erosion are clinically difficult to diagnose, since enamel is demineralized in a laminar manner without discernible softening of the surface. Vestibular erosion shows a silky-glazed, sometimes dull, surface in its initial stages, progressing into concavities and ridges. Concavities have a width that clearly exceeds the depth. Undulating borders of the lesion are possible. Initial lesions are located coronal from the enamel–cementum junction, with an intact enamel ridge along the gingival margin because marginal plaque serves as a barrier against acids and because the sulcular fluid has a neutralizing capacity.[2] Erosion on occlusal surfaces leads to rounded cusps, grooves, and restorations rising above the level of the adjacent tooth surfaces. In advanced stages, the entire occlusal morphology disappears. Laminar demineralization is characteristic for oral erosion, with a persisting enamel ridge at the crown margin (Figs 2-1 to 2-9).

Features of dental erosion
- silky-glazed to dull surface
- intact enamel along gingival margin
- restorations rising above the adjacent tooth surfaces
- altered morphology of the teeth.

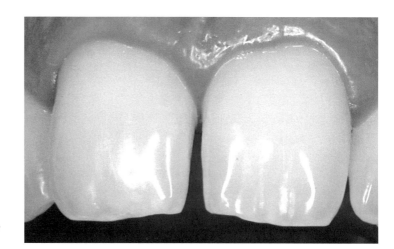

Fig 2-1   Initial vestibular erosions: the silky-glazed, sometimes dull, areas on the surface are typical.

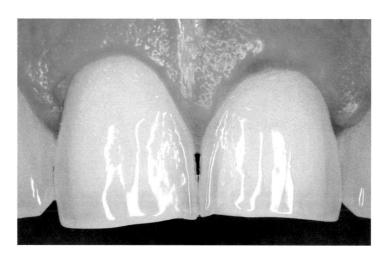

Fig 2-2   Early stage of vestibular erosions: distinctive surface defects are visible.

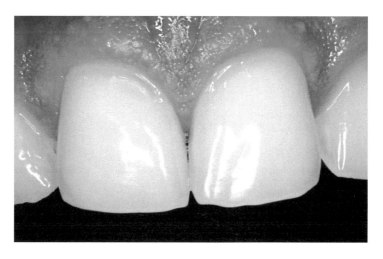

Fig 2-3   Advanced vestibular erosions. There is laminar loss of substance on the entire surface with a typically persisting cervical enamel ridge at the gingival margin.

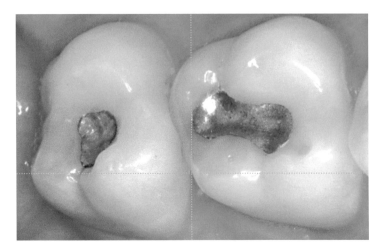

Fig 2-4 Initial occlusal erosion. Restoration overlap resulting from laminar loss of enamel.

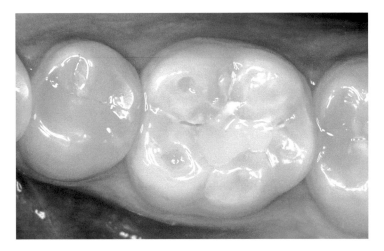

Fig 2-5 Intermediate stage of occlusal erosion: denting of cusps is clearly visible. Less than 50% of the tooth surface is affected.

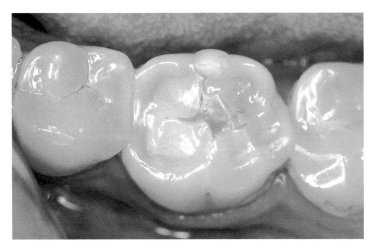

Fig 2-6 Advanced occlusal erosion with disappearance of entire surface morphology and expansive dentin exposure.

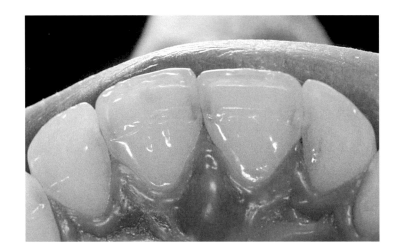

Fig 2-7 Initial oral erosion with laminar demineraliza-tion. Attritions are visible in the shape of ridges.

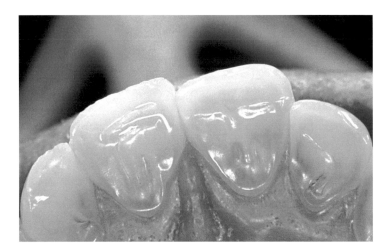

Fig 2-8 Advanced stage of oral erosion: the discolora-tions indicate an inactive stage.

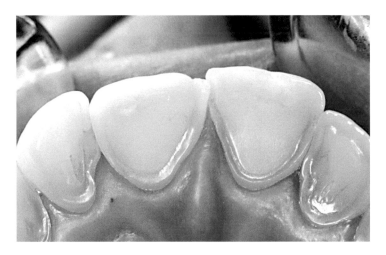

Fig 2-9 Advanced oral erosion with intact marginal enamel. Laminar exposure of dentin.

The location of erosive lesions can give indications as to the factors causing the damage. If acid damage occurs mainly on the palatal and occlusal surfaces, the action of endogenous acids is likely (eg vomiting). Asymmetrical erosions may indicate exposure to gastric acids through reflux during sleeping on one preferred side (see Chapter 4). Vestibular and occlusal damage can be observed with exogenous acids from foods and beverages.

Differential diagnosis

Dental erosion has to be distinguished from other enamel and dentin defects. It is possible for different defects to occur at the same time in a patient, such as caries lesions and erosions (Figs 2-10 to 2-12). However, it is pathophysiologically impossible for both defects to occur on the same tooth surface at the same time. Whereas caries is being caused by the biofilm plaque, erosion is created by direct acid exposure. Other tooth substance defects such as attritions and abrasions also have to be distinguished from erosions. Those mechanically caused defects mostly show sharp edges caused by physiological and/or pathological impact. An overlap of erosion, abrasion, and attrition is often found because of the increased susceptibility to damage that occurs in surfaces that have been altered by erosion (Figs 2-13 to 2-16).[3–5]

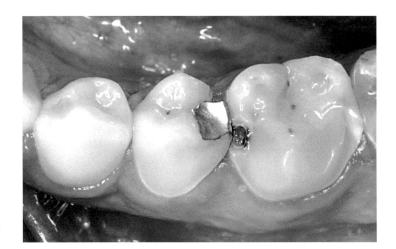

Fig 2-10   Distinctive vestibular erosions on teeth 35 and 36, open caries on tooth 36 mesially. Carious and erosive lesions may occur simultaneously, but never on the same surface at the same time.

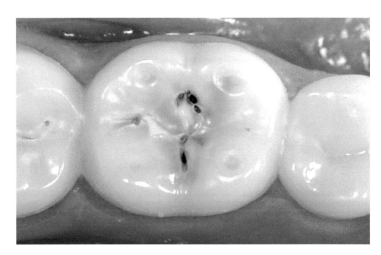

Fig 2-11   Occlusal surface of tooth 46: erosion and caries. There was first a period of erosive and then one of caries lesion formation.

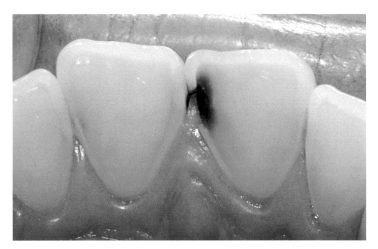

Fig 2-12   Oral tooth surface of maxillary incisors shows an advanced stage of erosions and interdental caries lesions.

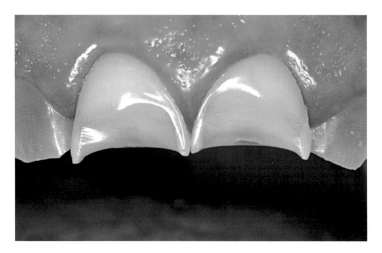

Fig 2-13 *Vestibular erosions and attritions: accelerated loss of tooth substance through mechanical impact.*

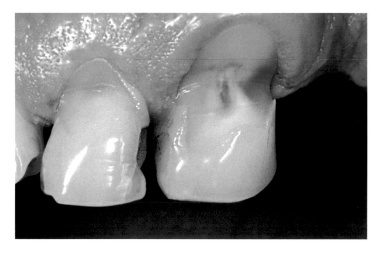

Fig 2-14 *Vestibular abrasive defects caused by inadequate toothbrushing technique. In contradistinction to erosive lesions, note the sharp edges. Often, striation caused by toothbrush bristles can be discerned.*

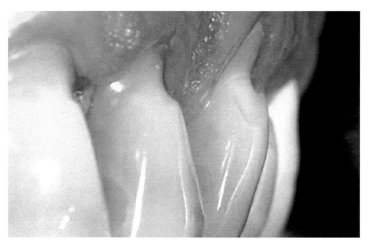

Fig 2-15 *Wedge-shaped defects are sharply confined. Often, an overlap of erosion and abrasion can be clinically observed.*

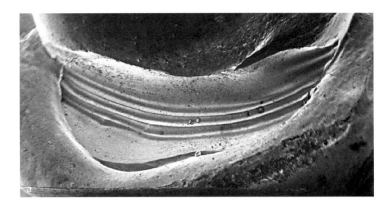

Fig 2-16a Scanning electron microscope image of a wedge-shaped defect. The sharp edges and striation caused by toothbrush bristles are clearly visible.

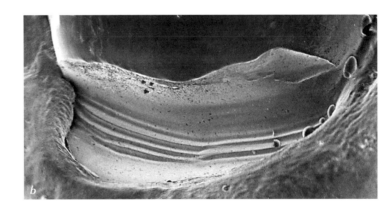

Fig 2-16b Same patient, 4 years later. Because of inadequate brushing techniques, the tooth substance has further deteriorated.

Basic erosive wear examination

When erosions are clinically observable or if an increased risk is indicated, the patient should be thoroughly examined. The BEWE is a short examination that efficiently allows erosions to be quantified (Tables 2-1 and 2-2).[1] BEWE allows the rapid detection and evaluation of acid defects. It is easy to use and offers recommendations regarding preventive and restorative measures (Table 2-3). With the exception of the third molars, teeth are being tested for acid damage vestibularly and occlusally, as well as orally.

The recommendations for ensuing treatment measures are only guidelines, as opinions differ considerably among experts, and social factors can play a role. Examples of patient treatments are given in Chapter 7. BEWE takes into account the entire loss of

Table 2-1   *BEWE: grading erosive wear*

Grade[a]	Clinical appearance
0	No erosive tooth wear
1	Initial loss of surface texture
2*	Distinct defect, hard tissue loss <50% of the surface area
3*	Hard tissue loss >50% of the surface area

[a]In grades 2 and 3 dentin is often involved.

Table 2-2   *BEWE assessment: in each sextant the highest grade value is marked and these are added to give a total score*

Highest grade 1. Sextant (17–14)	Highest grade 2. Sextant (13–23)	Highest grade 3. Sextant (24–27)	
Highest grade 6. Sextant (44–47)	Highest grade 5. Sextant (33–43)	Highest grade 4. Sextant (37–34)	Total score

Table 2-3   *Risk levels as a guide to clinical management*

Risk level	Cumulative score all sextants	Management
None	≤2	• Routine maintenance and observation • Repeat at 3-year intervals
Low	3–8	• Oral hygiene, dietary assessment, and advice • Routine maintenance and observation • Is reflux involved? Take photographs • Repeat every year
Medium	9–13	• As above • Identify the main etiological factor(s) for tissue loss and develop strategies to eliminate respective impacts • Fluoridation measures or other strategies to increase the resistance of tooth surfaces • Minimally invasive restorations; monitoring of erosive wear with study casts, photographs, or silicone impressions • Repeat at 6- to 12-month intervals
High	≥14	• As above • Particularly for severe progression, consider special care, which may involve restorations/reconstructions • Repeat at 6- to 12-month intervals

tooth surface material. Although dentin is frequently exposed in stages 2 and 3, BEWE does not generally include this when assessing severity as the irregularity of enamel thickness impedes direct correlation. Dentin is exposed considerably more rapidly in the neck of a tooth and in indentations. By excluding this factor, one potential source of error is eliminated and comparison of data collected by different examiners is facilitated. Moreover, the index can be applied with the patient present or with casts and photographic images.

The recommended time interval between examinations for the BEWE depends on the severity of the erosive lesions and on individual risk factors. Patients showing increased intrinsic and/or extrinsic acid exposure should be examined biannually. Generally, a time interval of 12 months or more is sufficient.

The examination is repeated for all teeth in a sextant but only the surface with the highest score is recorded for each sextant. Once all the sextants have been assessed, the sum of the scores is calculated (Table 2-2).

Clinical examples of the use of the BEWE

Case 1 (Fig 2-17)

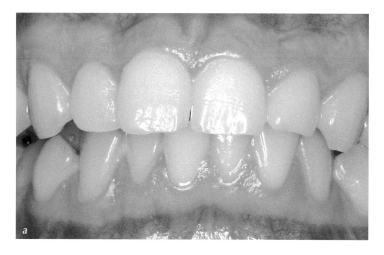

Fig 2-17a *Vestibular view (2nd and 5th sextant) indicates no substance loss:* **grade 0**.

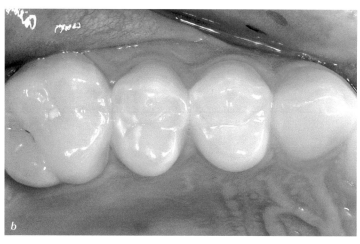

Fig 2-17b *Occlusal view of 1st sextant shows initial loss of surface structure:* **grade 1**.

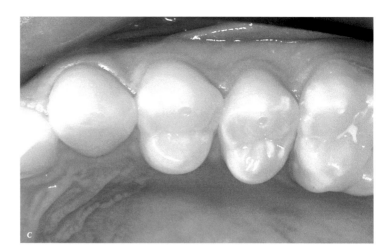

Fig 2-17c   *Occlusal view of 3rd sextant shows initial loss of surface structure:* **grade 1**.

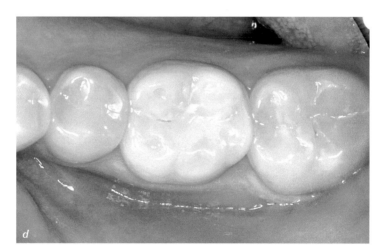

Fig 2-17d   *Occlusal view of 4th sextant shows a clearly visible loss of tooth substance (<50% of the surface area) on tooth 36:* **grade 2**.

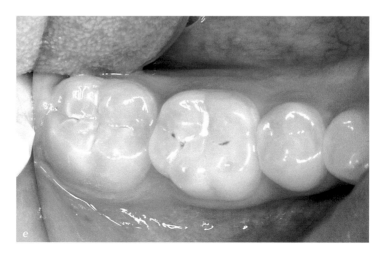

Fig 2-17e   *Occlusal view of 6th sextant shows a clearly visible loss of tooth substance (<50% of the surface area) on tooth 46:* **grade 2**.

BEWE scores			Case 1
1 1. Sextant (17–14)	**0** 2. Sextant (13–23)	**1** 3. Sextant (24–27)	
2 6. Sextant (44–47)	**0** 5. Sextant (33–43)	**2** 4. Sextant (37–34)	**6** Total score
➡ Degree of **severity** = **low**			

Case 2 (Fig 2-18)

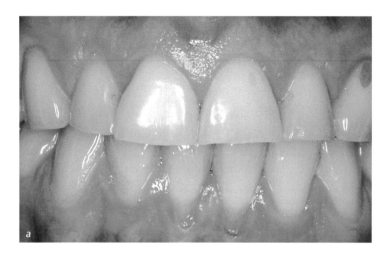

*Fig 2-18a   Vestibular view (2nd and 5th sextant) shows a clearly visible loss of tooth substance (<50% of the surface area): **grade 2**.*

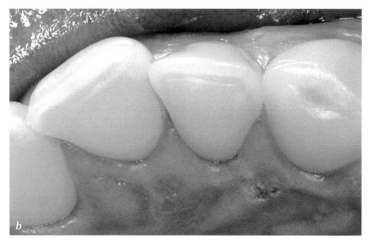

*Fig 2-18b   Detail of oral and incisal view (2nd sextant) shows a severe loss of tooth substance (≥50% of the surface area): **grade 3**.*

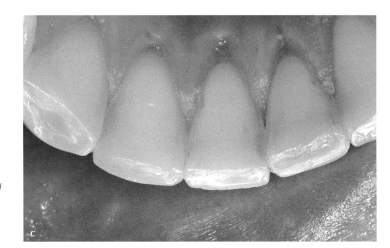

Fig 2-18c Detail of oral and incisal view (5th sextant) shows a loss of tooth substance (<50% of the surface area): **grade 2.**

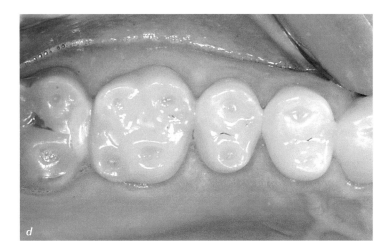

Fig 2-18d Severe loss of tooth substance on 1st sextant (≥50% of the surface area): **grade 3.**

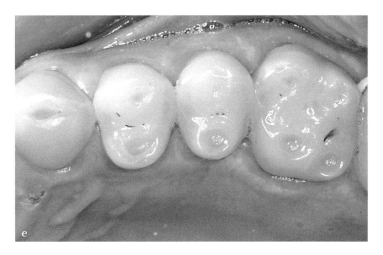

Fig 2-18e Loss of ≥50% of the surface area on 3rd sextant: **grade 3.**

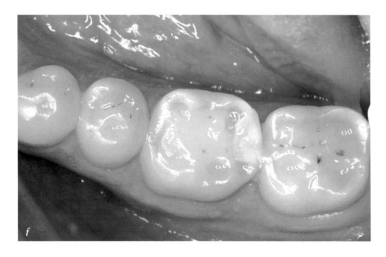

Fig 2-18f *Lesions in an advanced stage on the 4th sextant (≥50% of the surface area):* **grade 3.**

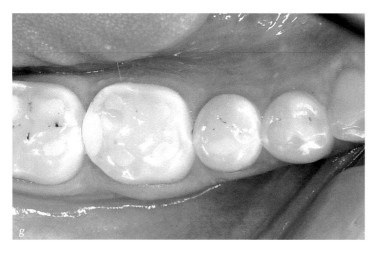

Fig 2-18g *Severe loss of tooth substance on the 6th sextant (≥50% of the surface area):* **grade 3.**

BEWE scores			Case 2
3	3	3	
1. Sextant (17–14)	2. Sextant (13–23)	3. Sextant (24–27)	
3	2	3	17
6. Sextant (44–47)	5. Sextant (33–43)	4. Sextant (37–34)	Total score
➡ Degree of **severity = high**			

Note: All tooth surfaces (vestibular, occlusal–incisal, oral) of all sextants have to be included for valid evaluation.

Chapter 3

Prevalence, incidence, and localization of erosion

Thomas Jaeggi and Adrian Lussi

Summary

The occurrence of dental erosion, as well as the severity of erosion when it occurs, has been increasing for several years now. It is, however, difficult to compare the various epidemiological studies, as evaluation methods as well as subject selection vary considerably. Studies on incidence are rare.[6–10] It appears that the prevalence of dental erosion is significantly higher in studies investigating younger subjects than in studies investigating older age groups. With increasing age, these currently younger patients have to expect further deterioration of their lesions. This indicates that, in the future, an increase of dental erosion in any age group has to be anticipated. Accordingly, preventive measures need to be initiated as early as possible to slow down the occurrence and progression rate of dental erosion. In this chapter, data on prevalence and incidence of dental erosion will be presented. The progression of lesions, and the areas affected, will be discussed using clinical case studies.

Prevalence of erosion

Various epidemiological studies have investigated the occurrence and degree of severity of dental erosion in specific age groups. The methods and indices used vary considerably, limiting the comparability of the results. One important difference is the number of teeth per person included in the evaluation. Whereas some studies included all teeth and tooth surfaces,[7,9,10–25] others included a selection of teeth only, for example anterior teeth and first molars.[6,26–39] Significantly more studies have investigated children and young adults than older demographic sections. Overall, this likely reflects the availability of data from school populations.

Table 3-1 *Prevalence of dental erosion according to age group*

Age group (years)	Affected people (%)
2–5	6–50
5–9	14 (permanent dentition)
9–17	11–100
18–88	4–82

Several studies with pre-school children (2 to 5 years of age) have indicated erosion in primary teeth in 6–50% of all children surveyed.[19,26,32,35] Wiegand et al[24] investigated 463 children aged 2–7 years. At least one tooth exhibiting signs of erosion was found in 32% of all subjects. Occurrence increased with increasing age: 23.8% of those aged 2–3 years were affected, 27.4% of 4 year olds, 30.4% of 5 year olds, and 39.5% of those aged 6–7 years.

Among children aged 5–9 years, 14% exhibited erosive lesions in permanent teeth.[15] In another group of children aged 5 to 15 years, lesions on permanent teeth were found in 25% and 68% of all the children exhibited at least one tooth with erosion.[34] Truin et al[36] also investigated children aged 12 years old in 2005 and compared them with results obtained 3 years earlier, in 2002. No change was found over the 3 year period in the occurrence of erosion (24%). Another study with children aged 12 to 14 years indicated a prevalence of 67%, 45%

of children showing low severity and 22% showing medium severity.[31] A study of children aged 13 and 14 years showed that 34% suffered from erosion in tooth enamel.[13] Summarizing results from studies investigating children aged 9 to 17 years led to prevalences between 11% and 100%.[6–8,10–12,14,17,20,23,27–29,37,38,40]

Studies with adults aged 18 to 88 years showed prevalences between 4% and 82%.[9,16,18,22,25,33] Table 3-1 shows the prevalence of dental erosion according to age group.

Incidence of erosion

Studies investigating the incidence of dental erosion are rare. Ganß et al[8] evaluated initial orthodontic casts made from 1000 children (mean age, 11.4 years). Five years later, the final orthodontic casts of 265 of these children were evaluated. Children suffering from erosion in their primary teeth showed a significantly increased risk for erosion in their permanent teeth (relative risk, 3.9). The number of moderate lesions in permanent teeth rose from 5.3% to 23% in 5 years; the number of children suffering from lesions in advanced stages rose from 0.4% to 1.5%.

A study with 622 children aged 10 to 12 years (mean, 11.9) showed dental erosion in 32.2%. Follow-up examinations after 1.5 years showed that the number of affected children had increased to 42.8%. The prevalence of distinct enamel erosion or with dentin involvement rose from 1.8% to 13.3%. Of the children not suffering from erosion in the first examination, 24.2% had developed erosion in the intervening 1.5 years. Erosion had progressed in 61% of those with lesions in the first examination, with increased depth of lesion and/or number of defects. Boys were affected more frequently than girls.[7]

Another study investigated 73 girls aged 12 years, 68% of whom showed erosion. After 1.5 years, 65 of the girls were re-examined. At this point, 95% of these girls suffered from erosive lesions and the number of affected teeth per child had risen from 2.2 to 5.6.[10]

Dugmore and Rock examined 1308 children aged 12 years and again 2 years later.[6] Incidence of erosion was 12.3%, with 56.3% showing erosion at age 12 and 64.1% at age 14. Severe enamel erosion increased from 4.9% to 13.1% in the 2 years, whereas the number with erosion affecting dentin rose from 2.4% to 8.7%.

> Erosion increases with age (number of affected persons as well as number of lesions). With advanced age, lesion progression increases.

Lussi and Schaffner[9] investigated the progression of erosion in adults, collecting data from 55 individuals at baseline and again after 6 years. Significant progression of erosion was found. Whereas 7% of the younger age group (26–30 years) showed occlusal erosion not affecting dentin in the first examination, this had risen to 25% after 6 years. Occlusal lesions affecting dentin rose from 3% to 8%. The older age group (46–50 years) initially showed 9% affected by enamel lesions, and 22% upon re-examination, whereas the lesions involving dentin damage rose from 8% to 26%. Vestibular lesions were less frequent but also increased over time in both age groups. Oral lesions were rare, did not show any progression, and were only observed in the older age group (Table 3-2).

Table 3-2   *Incidence of erosion*

Percentage of newly affected persons per year	
Aged 10–16	3–18
Percentage of persons with an increase in severity per year	
Aged 26–36	1
Aged 46–56	3

Case reports presenting the progression of erosion

The following section shows clinical cases with data spanning over several years. In every case, preventive measures were taken based on the estimated cause for acid damage. Consumption of acidic foods and beverages was reduced when necessary; endogenous factors were medicated. All patients showed normal salivation. Fluoridation was recommended to generate a protective calcium fluoride layer on tooth surfaces.

Case 1: Male patient, comparison of bitewing radiographs from 10 to 34 years of age (Fig 3-1)

Cause: Frequent consumption of orange juice, lemon juice, and fruit between 22 and 32 years of age, normal salivation. Areas showing distinctive progression are marked.

Fig 3-1

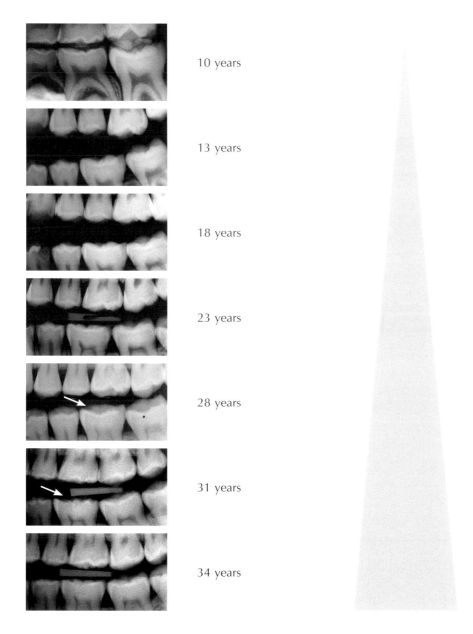

10 years

13 years

18 years

23 years

28 years

31 years

34 years

23

Case 2: Male patient, comparison of clinical situation from 21 to 23 years of age (Fig 3-2)

Cause: Moderate gastroesophageal reflux, no increased consumption of acidic foods or beverages, normal salivation. Areas showing distinctive progression are marked.

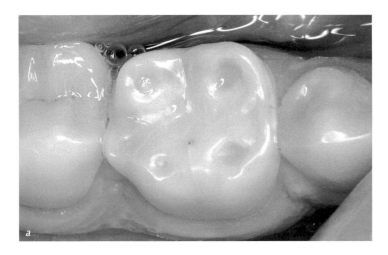

Fig 3-2a 21 years.

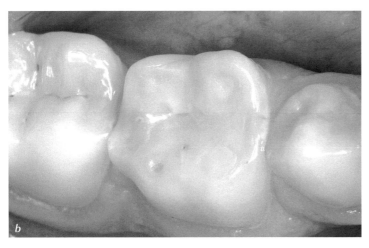

Fig 3-2b 21.5 years, erosion was treated locally with direct resin composite restoration.

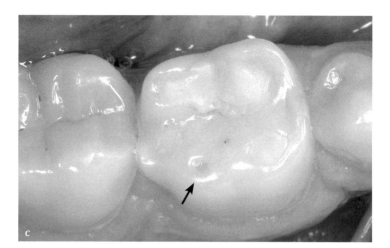

Fig 3-2c   *22 years.*

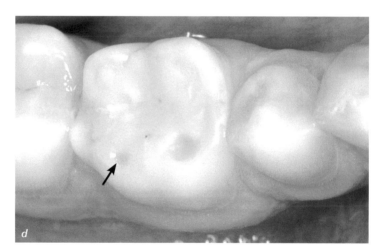

Fig 3-2d   *23 years.*

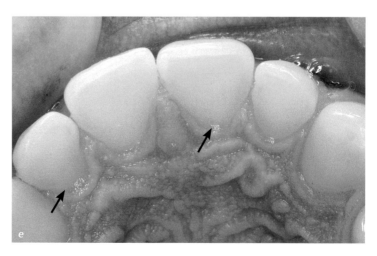

Fig 3-2e   *21 years.*

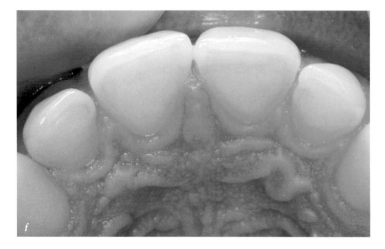

Fig 3-2f   *21.5 years.*

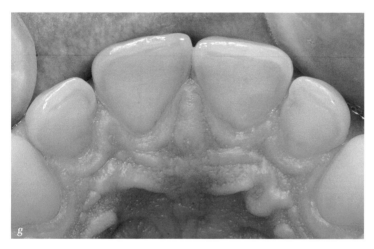

Fig 3-2g   *22 years.*

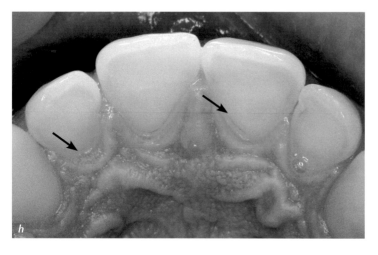

Fig 3-2h   *23 years.*

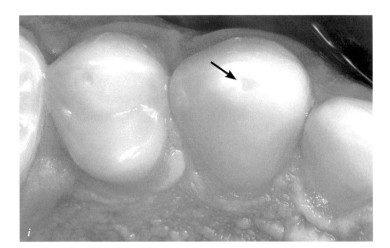

Fig 3-2i   *21 years.*

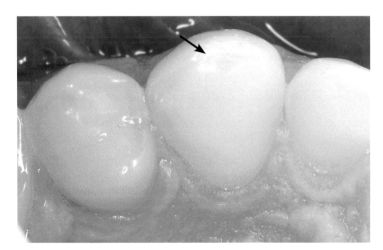

Fig 3-2j   *23 years.*

Case 3:   Male patient, comparison of clinical situation from 11 to 18 years of age (Fig 3-3)

Cause: Medicated for nightly gastroesophageal reflux, particularly aged 11 to 14 years. No increase in consumption of acidic foods or beverages, normal salivation. Areas showing distinctive progression are marked.

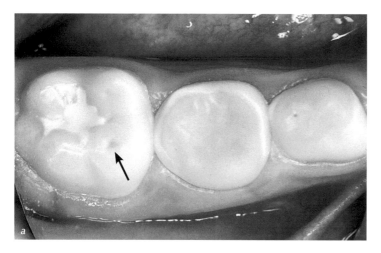

Fig 3-3a   *11 years.*

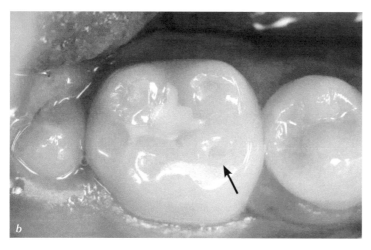

Fig 3-3b   *13 years.*

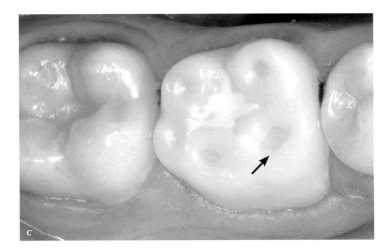

Fig 3-3c   *13.5 years.*

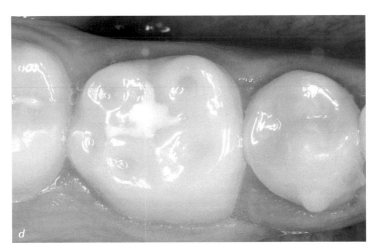

Fig 3-3d   *14 years.*

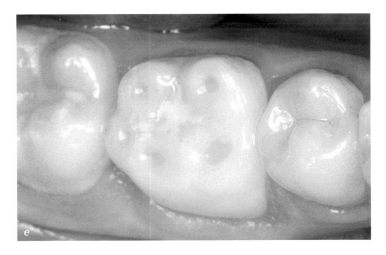

Fig 3-3e   *18 years.*

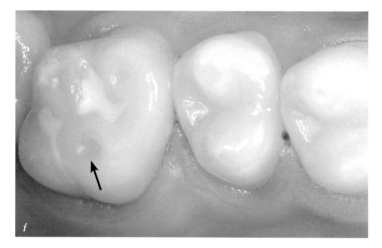

Fig 3-3f *13.5 years.*

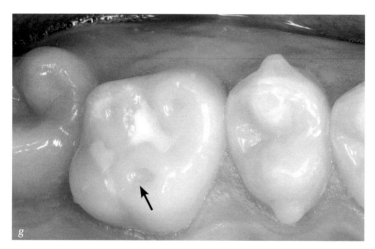

Fig 3-3g *14 years.*

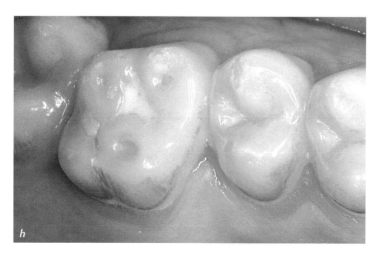

Fig 3-3h *18 years.*

Case 4: Male patient, comparison of clinical situation from 29 to 34 years of age (Fig 3-4)

Cause: Medicated for gastroesophageal reflux. Frequent consumption of acidic foods and beverages, normal salivation. Areas showing distinctive progression are marked.

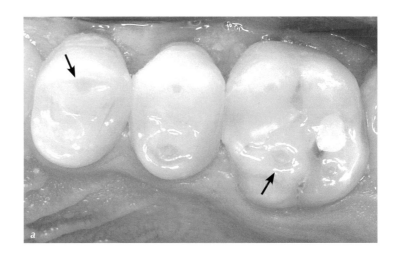

Fig 3-4a 29 years.

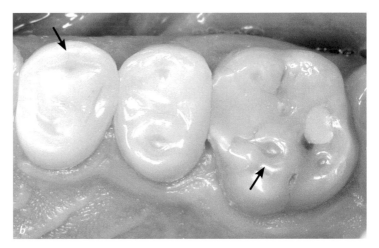

Fig 3-4b 34 years.

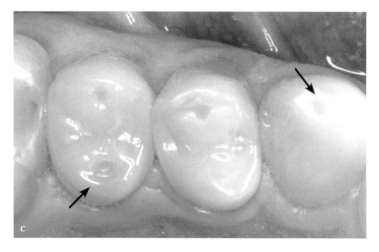

Fig 3-4c   *29 years.*

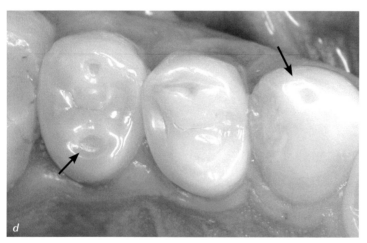

Fig 3-4d   *34 years.*

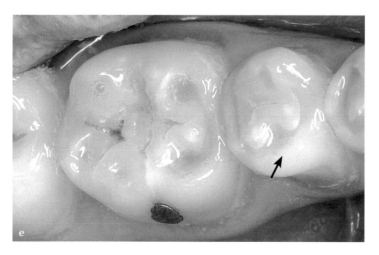

Fig 3-4e   *29 years.*

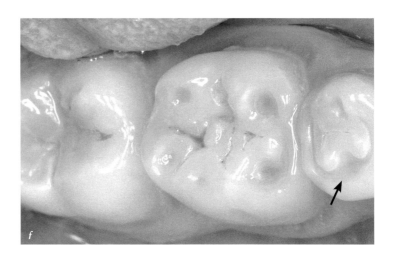

Fig 3-4f   *34 years.*

Locality of erosive lesions

This section discusses where erosive lesions occur in adults only; children and young adults are covered in Chapter 6.

Areas on tooth surfaces affected

Occlusal tooth surfaces are areas most affected by erosion in adults.[9,16,23,41] There are approximately four times more lesions here than on vestibular surfaces. Oral erosions are rare.[9]

Areas affected on specific teeth

Occlusal erosions are often found in molars of both jaws, with first molars of the mandible being affected most frequently. Vestibular erosions are most frequently found in the canine/premolar area of the maxilla as well as the mandible, followed by incisors of the maxilla, and molars in both jaws. The rarely occurring oral erosions are found on the tooth surfaces of maxillary incisors and canines (Figs 3-5 to 3-7).[9,16,18,41]

> **Frequency of dental erosion on tooth surfaces:**
> occlusal >> vestibular > oral

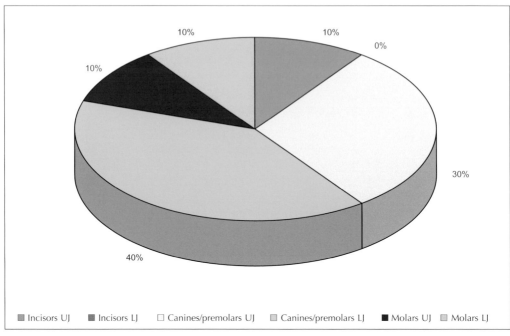

Fig 3-5 Distribution of vestibular erosions over the age range 18–63 years (UJ: maxilla; LJ: mandible).[9,16,18,41]

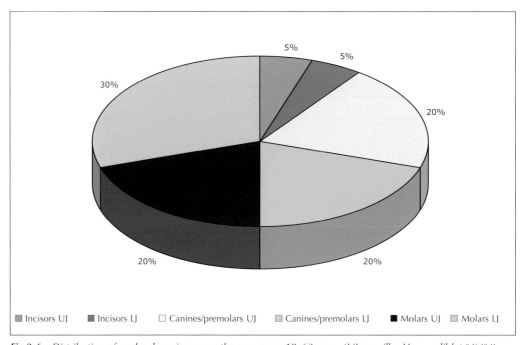

Fig 3-6 Distribution of occlusal erosions over the age range 18–63 years (UJ: maxilla; LJ: mandible).[9,16,18,41]

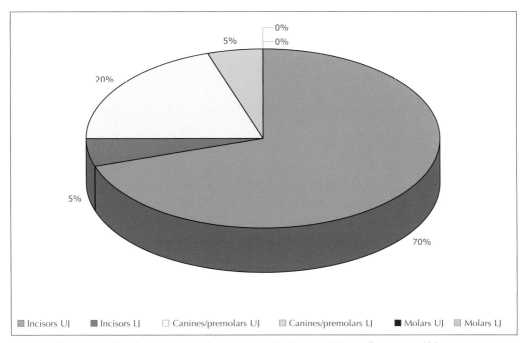

Fig 3-7 Distribution of oral erosions over the age range 18–63 years (UJ: maxilla; LJ: mandible).[9,16,18,41]

Frequency of dental erosion on teeth:

vestibular   canines/premolars (both jaws)
occlusal   molars (mandible)
oral   incisors (maxilla)

35

Chapter 4

Etiology and risk assessment

Adrian Lussi and Thomas Jaeggi

Summary

This chapter discusses various extrinsic and intrinsic factors leading to or preventing erosion. It will show that the degree of erosive potential of foodstuffs and beverages is not determined by the pH alone, but also by its interaction with other factors such as calcium, phosphate, fluoride content, type of acid, and buffering capacities. The relevant factors are grouped as patient-related, nutritional, and general factors.

Etiology

Dental erosion has multifactorial etiology. Protective and damaging factors have to be considered. Figure 4-1 shows an overview of patient-related and nutritional factors. These processes will be modified by other general factors represented in the outermost circle in the figure.

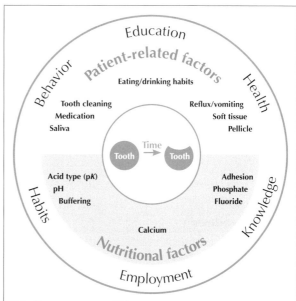

Fig 4-1   Factors influencing the occurrence of dental erosion.

Patient-related factors

Dietary habits

The manner of consumption of erosive foods and beverages (sipping, sucking, with/without straw) determines the duration and localization of acid exposure and, therefore, the appearance of dental erosion.[42–44] The frequency and duration of acidic exposure is significant in determining the amount of tooth decay, and these are vitally important to consider for preventive measures. Exposure to acid overnight can lead to more erosion because there is decreased saliva production during sleeping. For example, children drinking from baby bottles with acidic and/or sweet beverages during sleeping suffer not only from caries, but also from massive dental erosion.

Reflux and eating disorders

Gastroesophageal reflux disease

Gastroesophageal reflux disease (GERD) is a condition that develops when the reflux of stomach contents causes troublesome symptoms and/or complications. It can give rise to either esophageal or extraesophageal features. The definition used includes a patient-centered approach that is independent of endoscopic findings, subclassification of the disease into discrete syndromes, and recognition of laryngitis, cough, asthma, and dental erosions as possible GERD syndromes.[45]

The pH of the stomach contents varies with the types of food and drink consumed; however, the fasting pH is normally between 0.8 and 2.0. In addition to hydrochloric acid, the gastric juices contain enzymes such as pepsin as well as bile acids, which can influence erosion, particularly of dentin. Conditions increasing intra-abdominal pressure (eg, adiposity, constipation), hiatal hernia of the diaphragm, and sphincter relaxants (eg, nitrate, calcium channel blockers) predispose to GERD. GERD is one of the most frequently diagnosed gastroenterological problems, with equal prevalence in adults and children.[46–48] Approximately 7–10% of the population suffer from daily heartburn or acid regurgitation. Even 8% of children at the age of 1 year show reflux.[49]

> Gastroesophageal reflux occurs in approximately 10% of adults and children alike and often leads to erosive tooth damage.

Pathologically increased reflux does not always lead to symptoms. More than 50% of patients with reflux suffer from erosive damage of the esophageal mucosa (reflux esophagitis), but 40% of these patients with reflux esophagitis do not show reflux discomfort.[46,50–53] This indicates that reflux-related damage in the upper gastric system often occurs without typical symptoms. Characteristic symptoms for reflux are listed in Table 4-1.

Table 4-1 *Possible symptoms of gastroesophageal reflux*

- Dental erosions

- Acid regurgitation

- Heartburn

- Epigastric pain, particularlyy after certain foods and beverages (eg, wine, citric juices, vinegar, fatty foods, tomatoes, peppermint)

- Acidic or bitter taste after waking up

- Painful hiccups (odynophagia) or discomfort behind the breastbone (dysphagia)

- Nausea

- Vomiting

- Coughing

- Chronic respiratory symptoms (asthma, dyspnea)

When extrinsic factors can be excluded, intrinsic factors such as frequent vomiting and GERD reflux are suspected to cause dental erosions.

Often patients only notice their indisposition after teeth become hypersensitive. Other symptoms are stomach pains, burning or pain in the area of the esophagus/pharynx, or a sour/bitter taste in the mouth. Epigastric pain after the consumption of wine, citric foods and beverages, or fatty foods also indicates gastroesophageal reflux (Table 4-1). Since patients often consider their reflux normal, they have to be specifically asked, children as well as adults.

The main diagnostic courses of action are quantification of acidic gastroesophageal reflux and identification of an incompetent cardia or secondary damage caused by reflux. Acidic gastroesophageal reflux is assessed most reliably by ambulant 24-hour recording.[54–56] In this procedure, a small pH-testing probe is passed through the nose and down into the esophagus. The pH sensor is placed 5 cm above the cardia and will measure and record pH values over the course of 24 hours. Patients record any symptoms and/or dietary habits and these can be correlated with measurement of reflux. Gastroesophageal reflux with regurgitation during sleeping can lead to severe erosive lesions. Because of sleeping habits, such erosions are often distributed asymmetrically (Fig 4-2).

Asymmetric distribution of erosion points towards reflux during sleeping.

Bulimia and anorexia
Another patient-related risk factor where gastric juices can cause tooth erosion is the frequent vomiting that can form part of anorexia and bulimia

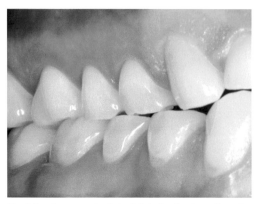 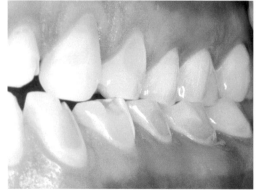

Fig 4-2 Asymmetric (left–right) distribution of erosion resulting from nightly reflux.

Table 4-2 Symptoms of frequent vomiting in bulimia/anorexia

- Dental erosion
- Enlargement of the parotid gland
- Redness in palate and pharynx
- Formation of rhagades on lips
- Changes in skin and nail of index and middle fingers
- Injuries/tooth marks on the back of the hand (sign of forced vomiting)

nervosa. Prevalence of bulimia nervosa with women aged 18–35 years is around 5% in western societies, with a rising tendency.[57] Most patients suffering from anorexia nervosa are between 12 and 20 years of age. Prevalence of anorexia in this age group is 2%. Diagnosis is often easy with severely underweight anorexic patients. Patients with bulimia, however, tend to be of average weight, making it likely for years to pass until the disorder is diagnosed. Chronic vomiting usually leads to erosion in the occlusal and oral tooth surfaces in the maxilla, particularly in the area of the incisors.[58–62]

Frequent symptoms with bulimic patients are oral and occlusal erosions in the maxilla, metabolic and partially painful enlargement of the parotid gland (sometimes of the submandibular gland), xerostomia, erythema in the palatal and pharyngeal mucosa, and painful redness and swelling of lips, including desquamation and formation of rhagades.[63] These symptoms and a corresponding medical/dietary history should alert the clinician to bulimic eating disorders (Table 4-2). Dentists are often the first medical professionals to identify the occurrence of bulimia. However, clinical experience shows that bulimia is not always associated with dental erosion. This may be because there is hypersalivation before vomiting.[64]

Saliva, pellicle, and drugs

Another salient factor in erosion is saliva. Saliva protects the teeth from acid through thinning, neutralization, reduction of enamel dissolution by calcium and phosphate ions, and pellicle formation.[9,65–71] Uneven distribution of pellicle can cause uneven distribution of erosion.[72] Teeth forming thicker pellicle (mandibular teeth lingually) show less erosion than teeth with thinner pellicle formation (maxilla, anterior teeth palatal). Additionally, acid clearance is better in the mandible.

Saliva production can be reduced by radiotherapy of the head and neck area, or by certain drugs. Among these are tranquilizers, anticholinergics, antihistamines, antiemetics, and parkinsonian medications. Patients with erosion should be questioned about their drug use and side-effects. The influence of drugs on saliva production is subject to great variation. Under certain circumstances, a change of medication can be indicated after consultation with the treating doctor. It has to be noted that prolonged and frequent contact of teeth with drugs of low pH can directly cause or accelerate dental erosion.

Tooth cleaning

Softened tooth enamel is susceptible to abrasion and attrition, leading to over-lapping occurrence of erosion, abrasion, and attrition (see Chapter 2). Without such softening, much less tooth substance is abraded during brushing of the teeth (Table 4-3).[73] Consequently, soft toothbrushes and low abrasive dentifrices are to be recommended to protect enamel and to protect soft tissues. It has been shown *in vitro* that the potential for abrasion on erosive enamel and dentin is higher with electric rather than hand toothbrushes,[74,75] a fact which should be considered when recommending precautionary measures.

Nutritional factors

Type of acid, pH, and buffering capacity

It has been known for quite some time that acidic foods and beverages can lead to softened tooth substance. The consumption of soft drinks and fruit juices in Europe is increasing continually and currently lies at 30% of non-alcoholic beverages consumed. For Germany or Switzerland, this equals a yearly amount of 200 L per person.[76] A study with 14-year-old children (209 boys, 209 girls) showed that 80% consumed soft drinks regularly. More than 10% consumed soft drinks more than three times per day. The erosive potential of foods and beverages is, however, not only determined by the frequency of consumption and the pH of the item; it is also affected by its buffering capacity, chelator properties, and other factors such as calcium or phosphate con-

Table 4-3 *Abrasion through toothbrushing (in vitro): after pellicle formation (2 hours), citric acid (1%, pH 3.6) was applied for 3 minutes and then the enamel was brushed for 15 seconds*[73]

Acid	Toothbrush	Abrasion (nm)
No dentifrice		
No acid	Soft	<2
No acid	Hard	<2
Acid	Soft	~30
Acid	Hard	~30
Dentifrice with low abrasivity		
No acid	Soft	<10
No acid	Hard	<10
Acid	Soft	~45
Acid	Hard	~45
Dentifrice with high abrasivity		
No acid	Soft	<10
No acid	Hard	<10
Acid	Soft	~70
Acid	Hard	~85

centration. For example, chelating properties of beverages can influence the erosive processes through interaction with saliva. Up to 32% of salivary calcium can be bound in calcium–chelator complexes formed by citric acid.[77]

Foods and beverages can show different erosive potentials despite having similar pH values. Higher buffering capacities in foods or beverages prolong the elevation of the pH in saliva (Table 4-4).

Calcium, phosphate, and fluoride content

The calcium content of foods and beverages is highly relevant. Immersion of enamel in calcium-enriched orange juice as available in retail showed no softening of the surface. This kind of orange juice (pH 4) can be recommended to patients prone to erosion. In contrast, non-enriched orange juice caused distinctive softening of enamel (Table 4-4). Yoghurt is another product with low pH (~4), leading not to softening but rather to hardening of the enamel. This is because of its high concentrations of calcium and phosphate, leading to saturation. The concentration of fluoride in foods and beverages also seems to show a protective effect.[78–80]

Isotonic drinks are often acidic and undersaturated in terms of calcium and phosphate in relation to enamel or dentin and, thus, can lead to erosion. Cal-

Table 4-4   *The pH values of foods and beverages, titratable acidity up to pH 7.0 ("buffer capacity"), and change in hardness in vitro (→, no softening or slight hardening; ↘, slight softening; ↘↘, distinctive softening) (modified from Lussi et al[85])*

	pH	Titratable acidity (mmol/l)	Change in hardness
Drinks (non-alcoholic)			
Carpe Diem Kombucha fresh	3.0	39	↘↘
Citro light	3.0	75	↘↘
Coca Cola	2.5	18	↘↘
Coca Cola light	2.6	19	↘↘
Coca Cola zero	2.8	10	↘↘
Fanta regular orange	2.7	52	↘↘
Henniez blue mineral water	7.7	-	→
Henniez red mineral water	6.1	4	→
Ice tea	3.0	26	↘↘
Ice Tea classic (Coop)	2.9	26	↘↘
Ice Tea lemon (Lipton)	3.0	24	↘↘
Ice Tea peach (Lipton)	2.9	21	↘↘
Valser mineral water (with gas)	5.6	13	→
Valser mineral water Viva, Lemon + herbs	3.3	40	↘↘
Orangina	3.4	59	↘↘
Pepsi Cola	2.4	19	↘↘
Pepsi light	2.8	15	↘↘
Red Bull	3.3	98	↘↘
Rivella blue	3.3	38	↘↘
Rivella green	3.2	44	↘↘
Rivella red	3.3	42	↘↘
Sinalco	3.1	36	↘↘
Schweppes	2.5	64	↘↘
Sprite	2.5	39	↘↘
Sprite light	2.9	62	↘↘
Sprite zero	3.2	40	↘↘
Sports drinks			
Gatorade	3.2	46	↘↘
Isostar	3.8	56	↘
Isostar orange	3.9	60	↘
Perform	3.9	34	→
Powerade	3.7	43	↘↘

	pH	Titratable acidity (mmol/l)	Change in hardness
Drinks (alcoholic)			
Bacardi Breezer orange	3.2	60	↘↘
Beer Carlsberg	4.2	18	→
Beer Corona	4.2	8.2	→
Beer Eichhof	4.0	18	→
Champagne Freixenet semi secco	3.0	78	↘↘
Cynar	4.0	6.0	→
Hooch lemon	2.8	67	↘↘
Smirnoff Ice vodka	3.1	50	↘↘
Wine 1 (red)	3.4	77	↘↘
Wine 2 (red)	3.7	63	↘
Wine 3 (red)	3.4	76	↘↘
Wine (white)	3.6	53	↘↘
Juices and fruits			
Apple juice	3.4	72	↘↘
Apple puree	3.4	89	↘↘
Apricot juice	3.3	317	↘↘
Beetroot juice	4.2	49	↘↘
Carrot juice	4.2	70	↘
Grapefruit juice	3.2	169	↘↘
Kiwi juice (fresh)	3.3	206	↘↘
Multivitamin juice	3.6	131	↘↘
Orange juice (fresh)	3.6	113	↘↘
Orange juice 1	3.7	109	↘↘
Orange juice 2	3.6	121	↘↘
Orange juice (with calcium)	4.0	110	→
Pineapple juice (fresh)	3.4	60	↘↘
Rhubarb	2.8	345	↘
Dairy products			
Buttermilk	4.7	32	→
Curdled milk	4.2	112	→
Milk	6.7	4.0	→
Whey	4.7	32	→
Yoghurt Kiwi Tropicana	4.0	124	→
Yoghurt drink orange	4.2	69	→
Yoghurt nature classic	3.9	120	→
Yoghurt orange	4.2	91	→
Yoghurt pineapple	3.9	114	→
Yoghurt Slimline	4.0	133	→
Yoghurt forrest berries	3.8	159	→
Yoghurt lemon	4.1	110	→

	pH	Titratable acidity (mmol/l)	Change in hardness
Coffee, tea			
Coffee	5.8	3	→
Rosehip	3.2	19	↘↘
Peppermint	7.5	-	→
Black tea	6.6	1.5	→
Forest berries	6.8	1.0	→
Medication			
Alca C fizzy tablet	4.2	53	↘
Alcacyl 500 (Novartis)	6.9	0.5	→
Alka-Seltzer fizzy tablet	6.2	14	↘
Aspirine-C (Bayer) fizzy tablet	5.5	28	↘
Berocca (Roche)	4.3	60	→
Fluimucil 200 fizzy tablet	4.7	20	↘
Neocitran	2.9	74	↘↘
SiccOral	5.4	2.5	↘
Vitamin C fizzy tablet, Actilife	3.9	93	↘↘
Vitamin C fizzy tablet, Streuli	3.6	85	↘↘
Miscellaneous			
Vinegar	3.2	741	↘↘
Salad dressing	3.6	210	↘↘
Salad dressing Thomy classic French	4.0	141	↘
Salad dressing Thomy light French	3.9	145	↘↘

cium-enriched, non-erosive isotonic drinks are available retail. Several studies showed a reduction of the erosive potential of isotonic drinks by adding calcium or phosphopeptide-stabilized amorphic calcium phosphate (CPP-ACP).[81–83] Non-flavored mineral water have been shown to have no harmful effects in other studies.[84]

Other than these erosive properties of foods and beverages, there are other factors that influence the adhesiveness of beverages to the tooth surface, which then affects the erosive potential.

Upon detection of erosions or signs of an increased risk of erosion, a detailed risk analysis should be performed with the patient.

A recent study analyzed 60 dietary substances and medications and showed that the pH, the buffer capacity, and the concentrations of fluoride and calcium were the variables with significant impact for dental erosion.[85]

General factors

Chemical industry

In the past, erosions were often connected with the work place. Even today, this possibility should still be included in a risk analysis. Regular contact with acids in the work place increases the occurrence and severity of dental erosions. A study that compared battery manufacturers with car mechanics in Ibadan, Nigeria, showed that 41% of battery workers had erosive tooth damage compared with 3% of car mechanics.[86] A study investigating the oral health of workers in the phosphate industry in Jordan had similar results; many erosive effects were found and 80% of workers suffered from tooth hypersensitivity.[87] The development of erosions caused by acidic fumes at the work place is well documented. There seems to be no difference between organic and inorganic acids in effects.

Tuominen and coworkers investigated the effect of organic and inorganic acidic fumes on teeth. Out of 169 workers participating in the study, 88 were exposed to acidic fumes and 81 served as control group. Prevalence of tooth substance loss was 63% in workers exposed to inorganic acidic fumes, 50% in those exposed to organic acidic fumes, and only 25% in the control group. Participants working with acid showed significantly more erosive defects in their maxilla than the control group, specifically in anterior teeth rather than posterior teeth.[88-90]

Another study investigated the correlation of acid concentration in the air at a German battery manufacturer and the prevalence and severity of erosive tooth damage.[91] Sulfuric acid in the atmosphere of the factory was 0.4–4.1 mg/cm^3. Erosions were found on anterior teeth only, while attrition occurred also in posterior teeth. Because of the high number of crown restorations, it was impossible to show a dose–effect relationship. The authors of the study considered that erosions caused by acidic fumes should be classified as an occupational disease.[91]

Westergaard et al investigated 425 employees of a pharmaceutical/biotechnology company, using 202 newly employed workers as a control group. No correlation between exposure to proteolytic enzymes and the occurrence of erosion could be found.[74]

In a systematic review of the literature, evidence for a higher risk of erosion from acid exposure in the work place could only be found in the battery-manufacturing and galvanizing industries.[92]

Wine industry and alcohol consumption

Wine may have an erosive potential because of its low pH and low concentration of calcium and phosphate (see Table 4-4). The number of professional wine tasters is increasing worldwide. Sweden and Finland employ wine tasters as consultants for state-owned wine shops and Swedish wine tasters test 20 to 50 different wines per week, on average. Wiktorsson et al investigated the prevalence and severity of erosion with 19 professional wine tasters, 14 of whom showed erosion, predominantly on the vestibular surfaces of the incisors and canines of the maxilla.[93] The severity of the lesions increased with the number of years in service. The authors concluded that dental erosion is an occupational risk for professional wine tasters. As a result, wine tasters employed with the Swedish Government were awarded preventive treatment free of charge.[93] Various case reports in connection with wine consumption have shown an increased risk of hypersensitivity and loss of tooth substance, illustrating the importance of early diagnosis and prophylaxis.[94–96]

Alcoholics often suffer from dental erosion. Although the direct influence of alcohol cannot be excluded, the main cause is gastroesophageal reflux, which explains the clinical appearance in these patients.

> Regular contact with inorganic and organic acids at the work place can favor the formation of dental erosions, or increase their severity. Professions with the highest occupational risk are workers in the chemical and wine industries.

Sport

Athletic activity leads to dehydration and athletes often consume sports drinks as well as energy drinks to ensure water and electrolyte balance. The erosive potential of sports drinks is generally known and is comparable to that of acidic soft drinks. It has to be noted that the consumption of sports drinks during exercise shows very little advantage over the consumption of water.[97] However, sports drinks are consumed in larger quantities than water, which facilitates the maintenance of water balance.[92,98] In consequence, this may be of relevance for athletic performance since frequently only around 50% of liquid loss is being compensated during physical exercise.[99] It is the responsibility of dental practitioners to inform athletes of the risk connected with the consumption of sports drinks.[100]

Some case reports have shown a correlation between physical activity and dental erosion. A study investigating 25 swimmers and 20 cyclists showed significantly more tooth substance loss among cyclists. However, no correlation could be shown between the consumption of sports drinks and the occurrence of dental erosion.[101]

A US study showed that 92% of the investigated athletes consumed sports drinks but only 37% suffered from erosion. No statistical evidence was found showing a correlation between dental erosion and the amount and frequency of consumption of sports drinks, nor did the duration of regular consumption or the consumption of sports drinks outside physical activity seem to have an effect.[102] The prevalence of erosion with these athletes was comparable to the one found in an epidemiological study with subjects chosen randomly from amongst the general population.[18] This further supports the assumption that non-excessive consumption of sports drinks does not increase the prevalence of dental erosion. An in-situ study showed comparable results between the erosive effects of sports drinks and that of mineral water. Consumption of sports drinks led to erosion with healthy test subjects, but to varied degrees.[103] Today, as mentioned above, non-erosive sports drinks with added calcium are available on the market.

In summary, the consumption of sports drinks can be a co-factor in the development and progression of erosive lesions. For proper erosions to be formed, other detrimental factors have also to be present.

Badly balanced pH values in water of swimming pools can be a potential reason for the development of dental erosion in regular swimmers. A survey showed increased prevalence for competitive swimmers performing intense training in chlorinated pool water with low pH values.[104] The pH recommended for swimming pools is 7.2 to 8.0. Training in water in this range, even if time in the water is extensive, will not lead to dental erosion.[38] However, pools with badly managed pH can lead to dental erosions of considerable ex-

tent very quickly. A case report from a swim team showed 39% of the members of the team suffered from erosion. The swimmers regularly trained in a pool with water pH values of 2.7, which equals a concentration of hydrogen ions 100 000 higher than recommended.[105]

Strenuous exercise can induce gastroesophageal reflux in normal subjects.[106] Because of decreased tone of the esophageal sphincter during strenuous exercise, the lower esophagus can be exposed to three times the normal level of gastric juices.[107] As described above, gastroesophageal reflux can lead to dental erosion if gastric juice frequently reaches the oral cavity.

> Practicing sports can lead to dental erosion mainly through consumption of erosive sports drinks, or through gastroesophageal reflux caused by vigorous exercise. In most cases, additional risk factors have to be present in order for erosion to develop.

Risk assessment

Case history

As with all patients, careful establishment of a case history is of paramount importance for a useful risk assessment. Factors to be taken into consideration for the assessment of risk fac-

Table 4-5   *Factors to evaluate during risk assessment of erosion*

Case history (medical, dental, dietary, behavioral)
• Ask for a record of dietary intake for at least 4 days, including a weekend
• Ask for risk factors not mentioned by the patient
• Assess intake of citrus fruit, other fruit, berries, fruit juices, sports drinks, sugared drinks, tea infusions, alcohol, alcopops, pickled vegetables, raw vegetables, salad dressing, etc
• Stomach problems: vomiting, sour taste, retrosternal pressure, signs of anorexia
• Drugs: tranquilizers, vitamins, antihistamines, effervescent tablets
• Dental hygiene: hardness of toothbrush, brushing habits (how? when? how often? how long?), abrasivity of dentifrice
• Radiation therapy in head area, salivary gland disease
Evaluation of non-carious tooth defects
• Erosion index (BEWE), abrasions, attritions
• Photographs, models (in order to determine progression)
Saliva analysis
• Salivary flow rates, buffer capacity

tors for dental erosion are not only stomach conditions, use of medication, physical activities, and brushing habits, but also a careful examination of dietary habits (Table 4-5). This applies particularly to patients where location as well as appearance of the erosions point to exogenous acid exposure. Patients should be asked to meticulously record any food or beverage intake over the course of 4 days. The period of observation should include a weekend, as dietary habits often differ from regular weekdays (see the example in Table 4-6). Subse-quently, the clinician analyses the data provided by the patient. If the number of acidic inputs is higher than four per day, and if at least one additional risk factor applies, there is an increased risk for the development of dental erosion.[108,109]

Case history
More than four acidic ingestions per day plus at least one additional risk factor = increased risk of dental erosion.

Table 4-6 Dietary habits

Questionnaire for dietary habits

1. Please remember to carry this questionnaire on you on four consecutive days. Do make sure to include a weekend.

2. Please note the time as well as a precise description of all of your food and beverage intakes (including snacks). Every intake is important irrespective of time or quantity.

   The following categories might help you to describe the quantities for
   (a) beverages/fluids   spoons, cups, glasses
   (b) bread   number of slices
   (c) sweets   number, kind
   (d) drugs   teaspoons.

3. Be honest! The more precise your record, the more useful and helpful your dentist's recommendations will be.

4. Please describe the manner as well as duration of your dental hygiene (eg, toothbrushing 2 min, flossing, fluoride mouth wash).

Example: Thursday, 15 December 2011

Time	Foods/beverages	Dental hygiene
08.00		Toothbrush 2 min
08.30	1/2 cup of cornflakes, milk, 2–3 biscuits, 1 glass of orange juice	
10.15	1 cup of coffee with sugar, 1 roll with marmalade	

Time	Foods/beverages	Dental hygiene
12.00	1 plate of pasta, 1 sausage, 1 glass of sparkling mineral water	
12.45		Toothbrush 2 min
15.15	1 apple, 1 cup of black tea with sugar	
18.00	2 slices of white bread, 4 slices of cheese, 1 glass of Coke (sipped)	
19.30	2 biscuits	
21.00	1 bar of chocolate, 2 glasses of orange juice	
23.05	2 glasses of white wine	Toothbrush 2 min

Evaluation (filled out by your dentist)

Frequency of **sugar intake**	Day 1	Day 2	Day 3	Day 4	Mean value
Meals	4				
Snacks	6				

Frequency intake of **erosive products**	Day 1	Day 2	Day 3	Day 4	Mean value
Meals	2				
Snacks	3				

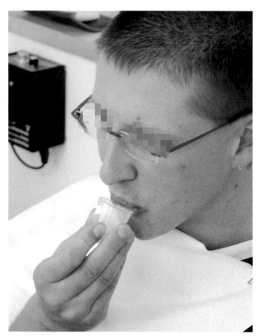

Fig 4-3 *Saliva collecting in the mouth is spat into a measuring cup to determine the salivary flow rate.*

Clinical examination

The inspection of the oral cavity includes all hard and soft tissues. The risk assessment for dental erosion should examine all the teeth for non-caries lesion-related tooth defects (erosion, abrasion, attrition). An index for dental erosion should be used (e.g. BEWE[1]). Photographs, study casts, and bitewing radiographs should be performed so that the clinical data can be compared over time. Monitoring and noting these clinical findings longitudinally is essential if the clinician is to be able to judge

the progression of dental erosion and, therefore, the success of initiated preventive measures.

Measuring salivary flow rate and buffer capacity

Decreased salivary flow rate and/or low salivary buffer capacity leads to an increased risk of erosion through delayed acid clearance. This, in turn, leads to longer exposure of dental surfaces to exogenous and/or endogenous acids. A simple way of determining these parameters is to measure the salivary flow rate and its buffer capacity. There are commercial tests available for this (eg, CRT buffer, Ivoclar Vivadent, Schaan, Liechtenstein; Dentobuff, Orion Diagnostica, Espoo, Finland; Saliva-Check buffer, GC Corporation, Tokyo, Japan).

Salivary flow rate is measured with the patient sitting in an upright position. The patient is asked to refrain from swallowing saliva, but rather to spit it into a measuring cup while time is being recorded for the patient to produce sufficient saliva (Fig 4-3). The flow rate of resting saliva is determined from the amount of saliva produced during this time. The flow rate of stimulated saliva is determined by the same procedure carried out while the patient is chewing on a piece of paraffin (Fig 4-4). Standard values of saliva flow rates are 0.25 ml/min for resting saliva and 1.00 ml/min or more for stimulated saliva.

Checklist for dental erosions

Diagnosis   BEWE (basic erosive wear examination)

Etiology

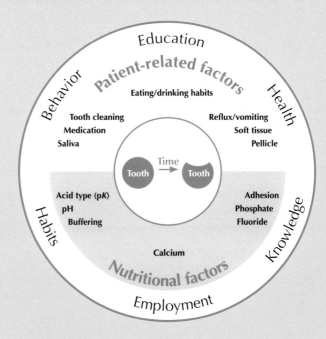

Risk assessment
- Dietary habits
- Frequency and amount of consumption
- Sports and occupational exposure
- Salivary flow rate
- Gastroesophageal reflux
- Bulimia and anorexia

Preventive measures
- Calcium content in foods and beverages
- Products containing (stannous) fluoride
- Changing traumatic tooth-cleaning habits
- Gastroenterological treatment
- Psychological treatment

Treatment
- Protection with bonding systems
- Resin composite
- Ceramic

Follow-up

For at least 1 hour prior to the measuring procedure, the patient should refrain from
- eating and drinking
- chewing gum
- smoking
- prophylactic measures (cleaning teeth, using mouthwash, etc).

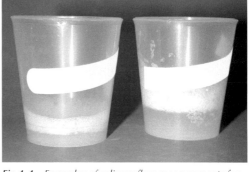

Fig 4-4 Examples of salivary flow measurements for resting saliva (left) and stimulated saliva (right).

Diagnosis of gastroesophageal reflux, anorexia, or bulimia nervosa

If the distribution and/or location of the erosions indicate influence of endogenous acids, the patient should be advised to see a gastroenterologist for a diagnostic assessment. In the case of suspected anorexia or bulimia nervosa, psychological assessment and treatment are indicated.

Patients suffering from gastroesophageal reflux are often unaware of their condition. Dental erosions are often the first visible symptoms.

➡ Gastroenterological diagnostic assessment is indicated.

Chapter 5

Prevention of erosion

Adrian Lussi, Elmar Hellwig, and Thomas Jaeggi

Summary

A prerequisite for preventive measures is to diagnose erosive tooth wear early and to evaluate the different etiological factors in order to identify persons at risk. In addition to precise questioning by the dentist, the patient should be asked to record their dietary intake for a distinct period of time. The clinician can then determine the erosive potential of the diet. Based on these analyses, an individually tailored preventive program may be suggested to the patients. It may comprise dietary advice, optimization of fluoride regimens, stimulation of salivary flow rate, use of buffering medicaments, and particular motivation for non-destructive toothbrushing habits with a low-abrasive dentifrice. Sealing of the exposed area can prevent further destruction and treat further dentin hypersensitivity.

Dietary habits

Once erosions are clinically visible, or there are signs of an increased risk of erosion, a detailed risk assessment should be performed with the patient. The various factors determining the risk for erosion as well as the methods for risk assessment have been discussed in Chapter 4. In many cases, a traditional interview is insufficient, as patients are often unaware of the level of their acid intake. An extended conversation with specific questions for the patient can provide information about the etiology of erosions. Furthermore, recording every food and beverage intake over the course of four consecutive days including a weekend can be of great use (see Chapter 4). Based on this information, preventive measures can be tailored to the specific needs of the individual patient. The data obtained from recording all foods and beverages consumed serve as a basis from which to reduce acid input and to change dietary habits accordingly. Consumption of acidic foods and beverages should be reduced and those that are taken should be consumed swiftly to reduce the time the products linger in the mouth. Sipping or sucking beverages through the teeth are habits leading to increased risk of erosion. As shown in Chapter 4, adding calcium, phosphate, and/or fluoride ions, or calcium phosphate complexes such as phosphopeptide-stabilized amorphic calcium phosphate (CPP-ACP), decreases the erosive potential of acidic beverages. Consuming modified beverages (eg, orange juice with added calcium, sports drinks containing calcium or casein) is a simple but effective measure to prevent dental erosion. Table 5-1 gives an overview of possible preventive measures to reduce tooth damage from consumption of erosive foods and beverages. Eating cheese can be recommended as another preventive measure. Cheese is high in calcium and phosphate and contains certain proteins showing protective properties. Acidic beverages are less erosive if cooled rather than consumed at room temperature.[110] Beverages and foods sweetened with xylitol may decrease the calcium loss in dentin and, therefore, seem to offer a certain degree of protection from erosion.[111]

Intrinsic acid exposure

In the case of intrinsic acid exposure (eg, with existing conditions such as anorexia/bulimia nervosa or gastroesophageal reflux), a causally determined systemic therapy should be initiated. Patients suffering from anorexia or bulimia require psychological or psychiatric treatment.

For patients suffering from gastroesophageal reflux, the focus lies on producing a detailed case history followed by recommendations for treatment (medications or, rarely, surgery). The best method currently available for treating reflux is to prevent it with the use of proton pump inhibitors (esomeprazole, lansoprazole, omeprazole, pantoprazole, rabeprazole), which raise the pH in the esophagus.[112–115] The necessary duration of antisecretory therapy in the case of dental erosion caused by reflux is not known. However, there are indications pointing to the possibility of discontinuing antisecretory therapy after a few years without relapse of reflux. Gastroesophageal reflux is an unstable condition, particularly with children, which is why a re-evaluation using 24-hour pH monitoring is indicated after 1 year.[48] If gastroesophageal reflux is severe and continuous, surgical measures might have to be considered. The most frequent surgical procedures are variations of gastric fundoplication, which can be performed laparoscopically. Long-term results of antisecretory therapy and fundoplication are comparable. However, a certain percentage of patients undergoing fundoplication also have to take antisecretory drugs. Furthermore, about 5% suffer from swallowing pain during the first few months after surgery.[116]

Table 5-2 is an overview of possible preventive measures for intrinsic acid exposure.

Table 5-1 *Recommended preventive measures for managing acid intake and reducing acid exposure*

Management of acid intake
• Reducing consumption of acidic foods and beverages to as few meals (and snacks) as possible

Reduction of acid exposure
• Avoiding sipping, drink beverages swiftly, no sucking between teeth
• Choose calcium-enriched (sports) drinks and foods, finish meals with cheese
• After acid consumption, rinse mouth with water, milk, or use (stannous) fluoride oral rinse
• Chew tooth-friendly gum to stimulate saliva production

Table 5-2 *Recommended preventive measures for intrinsic acid exposure*

Initiating therapy for the cause
• Suspected gastroesophageal reflux: referral to gastroenterologist
• Anorexia/bulimia: initiate psychological or psychiatric treatment

Simple measures to reduce erosion
• Avoiding reflux-inducing foods and beverages, eg, wine, citric acid, vinegar, fatty foods (full-fat, fried, etc), tomatoes, peppermint, coffee, black tea, carbonated drinks, chocolate
• Eating several small meals during the day, no large meal before sleeping
• Chewing (tooth-friendly) gum after meals to reduce postprandial reflux
• No toothbrushing after vomiting, rinse and clean tongue from acid remnants

Drug treatments
• Proton pump inhibitors such as esomeprazole, 20 mg 15 min before breakfast (in the morning if no breakfast is eaten) and 15 min before the evening meal

Surgical measures
• Surgery can be indicated for severe reflux (laparoscopic fundoplication); results are not necessarily superior to that with drug therapy

Dental hygiene

In addition to the measures discussed above, it is sensible to instruct patients suffering from active erosive lesions about adequate dental hygiene. Patients should be advised not to brush teeth immediately after acid exposure. The period of time elapsing between acidic intake and toothbrushing is sometimes recommended to be 30 minutes to 1 hour. However, in order for natural saliva to re-harden softened tooth substance sufficiently to withstand stress during toothbrushing, a considerably longer period of time than this is needed. It has to be stressed that, with respect to dental health, caries is still the main issue for most of the population. In many countries, caries prophylaxis quite correctly recommends toothbrushing immediately after meals. Instructing patients to wait 30 minutes to 1 hour after meals before brushing teeth is a problematic health-care policy, as it might result in people not brushing teeth at all. Therefore, the recommendation to leave a time interval before brushing is not recommended.

It is of paramount importance for health care personnel to recommend individual prophylactic measures and to monitor maintenance of these measures periodically. This enables encouragement for continuing these measures and the initiation of further preventive measures. Dentifrice with low abrasiveness, soft toothbrushes, and gentle toothbrushing techniques are indicated. The influence of the relative dentin abrasivity (RDA) and hardness of the toothbrush on eroded enamel has been discussed in Chapter 4. Toothbrushing before meals offers protection from caries and erosion.[117,118] Some researchers recommend avoiding brushing the teeth before acid intake because the brushing will destroy the protective pellicles. This can be avoided by using dentifrice of low abrasiveness, which leaves pellicle intact during brushing.[119]

> As a rule, teeth should be brushed immediately after eating. Other preventive measures (eg, toothbrushing and/or rinsing before acid intake) should be recommended only if erosive processes are present or vomiting occurs.

In this context, the availability of fluorides is relevant. Ganß et al[120] showed that regular fluoridation decreased the progression of erosion on human enamel and dentin *in vitro*. Samples of enamel and dentin were subjected to multiple cycles of de- and remineralization. Acid exposure was alternated with fluoride application and periods of remineralization. Enamel samples that were periodically treated with fluoride showed a significant reduction of erosive progression. The effect was even more prominent with dentin samples.[120]

Various studies have shown increased effectiveness of highly concentrated fluoride formulations if they were applied before rather than after the acid intake. Through precipitation of a calcium fluoride-like mineral, a protective layer is formed that leads to less erosive and abrasive damage. In conditions of decreased pH, this protective layer is decomposed before the underlying enamel is affected. To date, the question of the amount of time required for this calcium fluoride precipitate to be formed *in vivo* on healthy enamel has not been

Table 5-3 Recommended preventive measures by managing dental hygiene

- No toothbrushing immediately after acid exposure, fluoride prophylaxis prior to acid intake
- Using soft toothbrushes
- Using dentifrice of low abrasivity
- Using dentifrice containing fluoride
- Gentle toothbrushing technique
- Regular application of (stannous) fluoride oral rinse and/or highly concentrated fluoride gels

resolved. However, it has been shown that (1) the calcium fluoride-like mineral is formed very quickly *in vitro* and (2) that slightly acidic pH stimulates precipitation.[121] It should be mentioned that products for dental hygiene that are slightly acidic but contain fluoride show no erosive potential.[122]

Recent studies have shown that titanium fluoride (TiF_4) and stannous-containing substances also have protective properties.[123] While titanium fluoride can stain teeth, which is an undesirable side-effect, stannous compounds do not do this to the same degree. Stannous fluoride forms precipitates capable of withstanding acid exposure and consequently it protects teeth from erosion and/or its progression.[124] The assumption that dentifrice containing CPP-ACP (eg, Tooth Mousse) forms a layer protecting from erosion could not be confirmed in clinical studies.[125]

The application of fluoride or stannous-containing rinsing solutions before acid exposure is not always realistic (eg, before vomiting). However, it is possible to take prophylactic measures quite easily before going to bed as a means of protection from reflux during sleeping. It should be noted that wearing an empty mouthguard during sleeping is contraindicated for patients suffering from reflux. As a result of the capillary forces between mouthguard and the teeth, acidic fluids can enter the guard and effectively prolong the duration of acid exposure. This can be avoided by filling the mouthguard with a (neutral) dentifrice.

As mentioned in Chapter 4, radiation therapy of the head and neck can cause xerostomia or hyposalivation. This should be discussed with the attending physician in order to explore options of choosing a drug without side-effects that affect saliva production. Salivary flow rate can be augmented by chewing gum, leading to a reduction in postprandial reflux.[126] Tooth-friendly chewing gum should be chosen (Tables 5-1 and 5-2). Sour sweets or acidic saliva substitutes should not be recommended at all, but particularly not to patients suffering from xerostomia or hyposalivation as they lead to local erosions.[127,128] It has to be noted that some saliva substitutes currently on the market are acidic in nature. Table 5-3 shows an overview of recommended dental hygienic measures with erosion.

Table 5-4 *Application of adhesive systems as prophylactic measure*

- Use in the case of dentinal exposure and/or dentin hypersensitivity
- Has to be renewed every 6 to 9 months

Minimally invasive measures

Experience shows that patients refrain from seeing their dentists until suffering from dentin hypersensitivity. Once dentin has been exposed, adhesive systems offer a certain amount of protection from continued progression and can decrease the hypersensitivity of the teeth. It should be noted that this symptomatic "non-invasive" therapy has to be renewed every 6 to 9 months.[129]

Single-bottle systems or conventional bonding systems may be used (Table 5-4). Etching with phosphoric acid should be reduced to a minimum since the dentinal tubules are not obliterated. When using bonding systems featuring an acidic primer (eg, Syntac Classic, Optibond FL), phosphoric acid may be omitted altogether. When dentin hypersensitivity is the main problem, pastes containing arginine, potassium, or NovaMin may help. Further therapeutic measures (if possible) should only be initiated when the cause of the erosion has been determined and eliminated, and after the factors described in this chapter are under control. The success of preventive measures has to be monitored regularly. This is best accomplished with detailed photographs.

Chapter 6

Dental erosion in children

Thomas Jaeggi and Adrian Lussi

Summary

Dental erosion affects primary dentition as well as permanent teeth. The number affected and the severity increases with age. The pathophysiological processes in primary teeth are the same as those in permanent teeth. However, because of the smaller size and enamel thickness of primary teeth, severe lesions occur much more quickly.

The etiology of erosion in children is similar to that in adults: an increase in endogenous and/or exogenous acid exposure. In young adults, the two main factors are gastroesophageal reflux and immoderate consumption of acidic beverages. This chapter additionally discusses the clinical appearance of dental erosion and where it occurs in primary and mixed dentition.

Epidemiology

Several studies with pre-school children (2–5 years of age) showed that 6–50% suffered from erosion in primary teeth.[19,26,32,35] In one study, 32% of investigated children between 2 and 7 years of age suffered from erosion on at least one tooth, with the number of affected children increasing with age.[24]

Kazoullis et al studied children and young adults between 5 and 15 years of age.[34] The results showed that 68% suffered from erosion on at least one tooth. In this age group, children with primary dentition were affected approximately three times as often as those with permanent teeth.[31] In another study, 25% of the 814 12-year-old children investigated suffered from erosion. The comparison of these results with those obtained 3 years earlier showed no significant increase in erosive lesions in this group within the 3 years.[36] In contrast, El Aidi et al found an increase in prevalence of erosion.[7] They examined 622 children between 10 and 12 years of age (mean, 11.9); 32.2% showed erosion. This increased to 42.8% at the 18-month follow-up. Prevalence of distinctive erosion increased from 1.8% to 13.3% (see Chapter 3).[7]

Comparison of deciduous and permanent dentition

Erosive lesions caused by acid exposure can develop from the very first appearance of teeth in the mouth. Because primary teeth are smaller and have thinner enamel, dentin is affected much sooner, and lesions become severe much more quickly.

The literature shows conflicting results for comparisons of the rate of progression of lesions in primary and permanent teeth. Amaechi et al. found a rate of progression of enamel erosion in primary teeth exposed to orange juice that was 1.5 times that in permanent teeth.[72] However, another study found only minor differences in the susceptibility to erosion between primary and permanent teeth and other studies have confirmed these results.[2,40,130,131] Significant differences can be found in enamel hardness in primary and permanent teeth. On immersion of enamel samples in 2% citric acid (pH 2.1, 37°C) for 30 minutes, surface enamel softening was proportionate to the immersion time. Statistically significantly lower enamel hardness was found in primary teeth compared with permanent teeth initially and after acid exposure.[132]

It seems that the (probably) increased susceptibility to erosion of enamel in primary teeth does not occur in an initial phase of exposure. Only with increased time of immersion and/or increasing acid strength does the difference from permanent teeth become apparent. Additionally, it should be noted that primary teeth are more prone to abrasion because of their lower enamel hardness.[133] The effect of heightened loss of substance in primary teeth is frequently observed clinically. The interaction of erosion, attrition, and abrasion leads to more distinctive lesions in primary than in permanent teeth.

Etiology

As discussed in Chapter 4, dental erosion has a multifactorial etiology including both exogenous and endogenous factors. Regular and frequent consumption of erosive foods and beverages has to be considered the most relevant exogenous factor. The Union of European Beverages Association reported a constant increase in consumption of carbonated drinks and juices, as well as other non-alcoholic beverages such as sports and energy drinks.[76] Drinks of this sort, mostly of an acidic nature, are an important factor in the formation of dental erosion, particularly because of their popularity with children and young adults. The manner of consumption of erosive foods and beverages (sipping, sucking, with/without straw) determines the duration and locality of acid exposure and, therefore, the appearance of erosion. With respect to endogenous factors, gastroesophageal reflux seems to be of some importance for the formation of dental erosion in children.[134–136]

The presence of dental erosion in primary dentition significantly increases the risk of suffering from erosion in permanent dentition. The risk of permanent dentition being affected by loss of substance, which increases with age, can be prevented by early prophylactic measures.

Areas affected by erosion in children and adolescents

Generally, all tooth surfaces of the primary and mixed dentition can be affected by erosion. Millward et al investigated 178 children aged 4 years and found indications for erosive defects in almost half of them. The lesions were most pronounced on the oral surfaces of the incisors of the maxilla.[19] In another study, 42 children between 5 and 9 years of age were tested; all suffered from erosions, most of them on the occlusal surfaces.[15]

Ganß et al examined 1000 initial orthodontic casts of children's dentition (mean age, 11.4 years; SD, 3.3) for dental erosion. Erosive lesions could be seen in primary teeth in 73.6%, particularly on occlusal and incisal surfaces of molars and canines, and 11.6% had affected permanent teeth, particularly in the first molars of the mandible.[8] Figure 6-1 summarizes the distribution of erosions in primary dentition in various studies.[8,15,19]

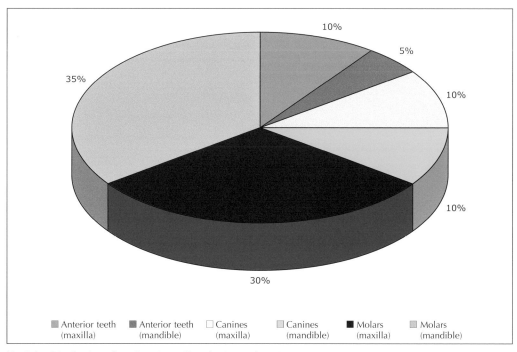

■ Anterior teeth (maxilla)   ■ Anterior teeth (mandible)   ☐ Canines (maxilla)   ☐ Canines (mandible)   ■ Molars (maxilla)   ☐ Molars (mandible)

Fig 6-1   *Distribution of erosions in studies of primary dentition.[8,15,19]*

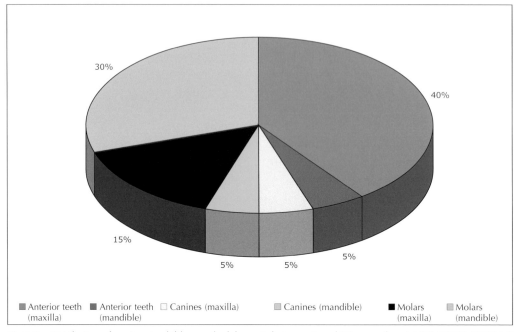

30%

40%

15%

5%   5%   5%

| ■ Anterior teeth (maxilla) | ■ Anterior teeth (mandible) | □ Canines (maxilla) | ▨ Canines (mandible) | ■ Molars (maxilla) | ▨ Molars (mandible) |

Fig 6-2 *Distribution of erosions in children and adolescents between 8 and 17 years of age.*[6–8,10–14,17,18,20,23,27–29,37,38,40]

El Aidi et al found erosive lesions in 32.2% of 622 children between 10 and 12 years of age.[7] The occlusal surfaces of the molars (teeth 36 and 46) and the oral surfaces of the maxillary incisors were particularly affected. The follow-up after 18 months showed even more pronounced erosion. Particularly teeth 13 to 23 showed a larger number of defects, and teeth 36 and 46 showed both more as well as more-severe erosion.[7]

Another study, investigating 458 adolescents between 13 and 14 years of age, also found a third affected by dental erosion, mostly on the oral surfaces of the maxillary incisors.[13] Milosevic et al studied 1035 adolescents (mean age 14 years) and detected erosion mostly on the occlusal surfaces of the first molars in the mandible and the oral surfaces of the maxillary incisors.[20] Al-Dlaigan et al examined 418 children aged 14 years and found that every one suffered from erosion, with minor erosions found on all tooth surfaces, moderate erosions on incisal edges of anterior teeth, and severe erosion on the vestibular surfaces of the anterior teeth.[11]

Examining two different age groups (345 aged 10–13 years and 400 aged 15–16 years), another study found most lesions in first molars and maxillary incisors.[23] Larsen et al investigated 558 young adults between 15 and 17 years of age, 14% of whom suffered from erosion on more than three surfaces, mostly orally on the maxillary incisors.[17] Figure 6-2 summarizes the distribution of erosions in adolescents between 8 and 17 years of age in various studies.[6–8,10–14,17,18,20,23,27–29,37,38,40]

Clinical appearance

The initial stages of dental erosion are difficult to diagnose for both primary and permanent teeth because surface demineralization of enamel does not result in discernible surface softening. Vestibular erosions have a silky or dull surface appearance initially, progressing into indentations and ridges in the enamel. Affected dentin often has a persisting marginal enamel ridge. As on permanent teeth, occlusally, rounded cusps are formed with bowl-shaped defects into the dentin. At a later stage, the surface morphology completely disappears. Oral erosions mainly occur in the maxillary incisors (Figs 6-3 and 6-4).[49,68]

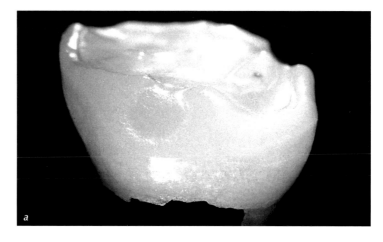

Fig 6-3a *Exfoliated primary molar, vestibular view. A typical advanced stage erosion is visible occlusally, with complete disappearance of surface morphology and extensive dentin exposure. There are pronounced indentations, a rounded enamel surface, and no sharp edges.*

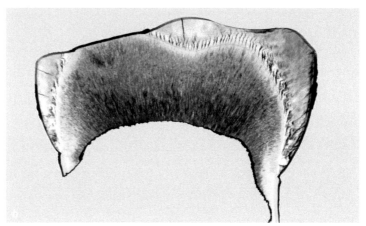

Fig 6-3b *The molar in histologic cross-section. The morphology of the crown is rounded and presents no sharp edges. Affected dentin is clearly visible.*

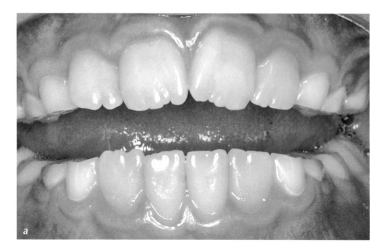

Fig 6-4a *Frontal view of mixed dentition. Deciduous teeth show considerable erosive substance loss.*

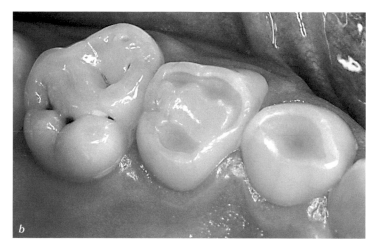

Fig 6-4b *In the 1st quadrant for the same patient, there is severe loss of substance affecting teeth 53 and 54 incisally and occlusally; tooth 55 is less affected, merely showing initial loss of surface structure. The basic erosive wear examination (BEWE; see Chapter 2) for the 1st and 2nd sextants is grade 3.*

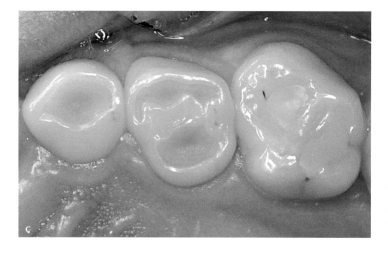

Fig 6-4c *A similar clinical image is seen in the 2nd quadrant in this patient. The 2nd and 3rd sextants both are BEWE grade 3.*

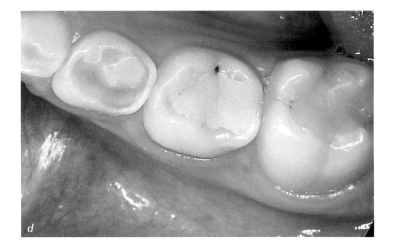

Fig 6-4d The situation is practically identical in the 3rd quadrant. Again, teeth 3 to 5 are affected. Another typical feature of erosion is the overlapping edges of the resin composite filling, which occurs because it has greater acid resistance than enamel (Chapter 7).

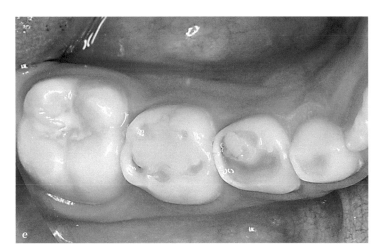

Fig 6-4e The 4th quadrant shows similar features, with clearly visible advanced erosions in teeth 83, 84, and 85. There is characteristic cupping and loss of surface morphology with affected dentin in all three teeth.

Restorative and reconstructive treatment of erosions

Thomas Jaeggi and Adrian Lussi

Case reports by
Carola Imfeld, Zurich;
Nadine Schlueter, Giessen;
Patrick R. Schmidlin, Olivier O. Schicht, Thomas Attin, Zurich;
and Anne Grüninger, Bern

Summary

When dental erosion is advanced, restorative or reconstructive measures become necessary. Before adhesive systems were available in dental practice, teeth with large erosive lesions could only be treated with crowns and fixed dental prostheses or removable dentures. Improved resin composites and adhesives enabled less invasive restoration of dental erosion. Nevertheless, teeth with severe erosive defects require the use of veneers, overlays, and crowns even today. Before invasive treatment can be carried out, it is necessary to determine the possible causes for erosion in order to initiate preventive measures to stop or slow down the process, which is essential for effective restorative treatment.

This chapter provides an overview of the durability and longevity of restorative materials in an acidic environment. Various treatment strategies are discussed, from minimally invasive direct resin composite restorations to complex ceramic reconstructions. Case reports by various dentists at university clinics present different solutions.

It should be considered a general rule that rehabilitation of erosive dentition should be as minimally invasive as possible, and preventive measures should be an integral part of therapy in order to protect the remaining tooth substance.

Longevity of restorative materials in an acidic environment

Successful use of adhesive systems is dependent upon the condition of tooth substance, which must be clinically evaluated. Bonding systems perform better on healthy, normal dentin surfaces than on sclerotic and cervical dentin areas, where blocking of dentinal tubules prevents adhesives from forming the plugs essential for a firm bond.[137] Ogata et al studied the effect of tubule orientation on the cohesion value of adhesives on dentin. Several adhesives showed better cohesion values on surfaces with parallel tubule orientation rather than those cut perpendicularly.[138] Another study investigated the effect of preparatory measures on the adhesive power of a self-etching adhesive system. Surface preparation with steel burs showed better results than using diamond burs.[139]

Adhesive values on dentin depend (among other factors) on:
- the number of cut dentin tubuli
- the diameter of dentin tubuli (degree of scleroses)
- orientation of tubuli cut
- surface preparation of dentin.

Recommendation: sclerotized dentin should be prepared with steel burs before etching. With open dentin tubuli and dentin hypersensitivity, etching time should be shorter.

Longevity of restorative materials

The longevity of dental restorations depends on the durability of the material and its wear resistance,[140] the durability of the interface between tooth substance and restoration, and the degree of tooth destruction, both the area affected and the level of stress exposure.

Several studies have shown good long-term results for restorative materials such as glass-ionomer cements and resin composites if applied correctly. A survival rate of more than 75% after 10 years has been shown for these filling materials if they are used for suitable indications.[141–143] When loss of tooth substance is more substantial and affects tooth structure, full ceramic restorations such as inlays, overlays, and crowns become necessary. Extensive research has been performed on the Cerec system, which showed good longevity rates of 90% after 10 years in several studies.[144–146] Improved preparation techniques, adhesive systems, and restoration materials enable increasingly small-scale restoration, which improves the lifetime of the restoration even if it is exposed to high mechanical stress.[147] It should be noted that the research described here examined posterior restoration to treat mostly caries lesions rather than erosion.

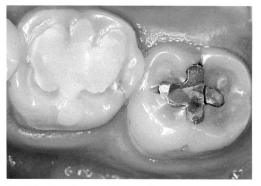

Fig 7-1 *Overlapping fillings with amalgam as well as resin composite and advanced occlusal erosions on teeth 37 and 36, showing the better resistance to acid exposure of filling materials compared with tooth substance.*

Longevity rate of restoration materials after 10 years:
- glass-ionomer cements
  (cervical fillings):   80%
- resin composite
  (lateral teeth):   75–80%
- ceramic
  (Cerec, lateral teeth):   90%

Chemical and physical alterations in restoration materials

It must be expected that an acidic environment will affect not only tooth substance, but also restoration materials in the oral cavity. Clinical experience, however, shows that changes to restorations occur on a much smaller scale than those in enamel and dentin, an effect which is illustrated by overlapping edges of fillings (Fig 7-1).

The chemical and physical alterations in tooth substance and restoration materials have been investigated in several studies. There are various methods of evaluating erosion of dental material: (1) testing dissolution properties, (2) residual weight measurement of a solution in which the dental material is immersed, and (3) measuring surface loss of a cavity filled with the material under investigation.[148] Materials are predominantly exposed to buffered and non-buffered acids and other substances (foods, beverages, food-simulating agents). Well-researched materials are zinc phosphate cements, polycarboxylate cements, glass-ionomer cements, resin composite cements, modified glass-ionomer cements, com-

Table 7-1 *Studies investigating the resistance to abrasion or surface substance loss of restoration materials after immersion in various media*

Materials	Media	Results
Ceramic	Coca Cola	Decrease in resistance to abrasion (Duceram > Vita Mark II)[149]
Polycarboxylate cement, zinc phosphate cement, GIC	Lactic acid, lactic acid–sodium lactate buffer	More substance loss with buffer solution (polycarboxylate > zinc phosphate > GIC)[148]
Resin composite, modified GIC, GIC	Different media with pH 1.2–7.0	Acid and abrasion resistance of material > enamel (Z100 > Fuji II LC > Fuji IX)[150]

GIC, glass-ionomer cement.

pomers, resin composites, and ceramics. All studies found that all materials were altered in acid environments. In terms of resistance to abrasion and loss of substance, ceramics and resin composites showed the best results, followed by modified glass-ionomer cements and conventional glass-ionomer cements (Table 7-1). A similar picture emerges when studying alterations in hardness of the materials under the influence of acid, with results depending on the type of the materials as well as the pH and type of acid forming the immersion media. It is interesting to note that materials reacted sometimes in ways other than what was expected (eg, increase in surface hardness with acid exposure) (Table 7-2). Studies investigating surface roughness also found best results with ceramics and resin composites, with least increase in surface roughness (Table 7-3).

Performance of restoration materials in acidic environments:
All materials show alterations with time. The most frequently occurring alterations were:
• increase in surface roughness
• decrease in surface hardness
• loss of substance.

Ceramics and resin composites showed better acid resistance and should be preferred to compomers and glass-ionomer cements in patients with dental erosion.

Table 7-2 *Studies investigating the surface hardness changes in restoration materials after immersion in various media*

Materials	Media	Results
Resin composite (Ariston, Silux, Z100, Surefil)	Saliva, water, citric acid, lactic acid, heptane, alcohol	Correlation between surface hardness change and substance loss; hardness change for all tested resin composites (increase/decrease)[151]
GIC, modified GIC, compomer	Coca Cola, apple juice, orange juice	Decrease in surface hardness after immersion in all beverages (GIC > modified GIC/compomer)[152]
Resin composite, GIC, modified GIC, compomer	Lactic acid, phosphoric acid, citric acid, acetic acid	Hardness change depends on the material and on pH and type of acid of the immersion solution (increase/decrease)[153]
Resin composite, compomer, giomer	Buffered citric acid solution (pH 2.5–7.0)	Decrease in surface hardness (compomer/giomer > resin composite); pH dependent[154]
Resin composite, GIC, modified GIC, compomer	Coca Cola, orange juice, sports drinks, yoghurt, soup	Decrease in surface hardness with Coca Cola (resin composite, modified GIC)[155]
Resin composite, GIC, modified GIC, amalgam	Saliva, Coca Cola *in vitro/in situ* (cycling)	No differences between materials; decrease in surface hardness for all materials with Cola (only *in vitro*)[156,157]

GIC, glass-ionomer cement.

Table 7-3 *Studies investigating the surface roughness of restoration materials after immersion in various media*

Materials	Media	Results
Resin composite, modified GIC, compomer	Water, saliva, pH cycling	Increase in surface roughness of all materials after pH cycling[158]
Resin composite, compomer, giomer, GIC	Water, citric acid (pH 2.0–6.0)	Surface roughness (GIC > compomer/giomer > resin composite); pH dependent[159]
Resin composite cement, resin composite, ceramic	Toothbrush abrasion with/without pH cycling	Surface roughness (Variolink II < Enforce/Rely X; ceramic < resin composite < resin composite cement); pH cycling without impact[160]

GIC, glass-ionomer cement.

Treatment strategies

Erosive loss of tooth substance is initially restricted to enamel. At this stage, no hypersensitivity occurs, and restorations are necessary only for esthetic reasons or to impede progression.

At an advanced stage, dentin is exposed. Reasons for treatment at this stage can be many: (1) hypersensitivity of exposed dentin, (2) impeded functionality of the tooth, (3) esthetic disfigurement, and (4) danger of exposed pulp as a result of advanced erosion.[161]

Conditions necessitating treatment:
- dentin hypersensitivity
- loss of functionality
- disfigurement
- danger of pulp damage.

Treatment should be minimally invasive. Adhesive materials are to be preferred in such a conservative treatment approach.[162] Healthy tooth substance has to be protected. Modern therapeutic measures adapt restoration to teeth and not vice versa. Difficulties can arise when the alveolar process and surrounding tissue compensate lost tooth substance (compensatory growth of alveolar crest).[163] Despite displaying massive loss of crown height clinically, occlusal contact is maintained, which results in space constrictions. In order to avoid invasive therapy, orthodontic measures can be expedient to create interocclusal space. Situations like these arise if compensatory shifting occurs with a whole group of teeth (eg, the anterior segment). Orthodontic measures might include fixed or removable devices (eg, Dahl device;[163] see Case reports 1, 7, and 8). After orthodontic treatment, erosively damaged teeth can be reconstructed.[164] Until a few years ago, heavily damaged teeth could only be treated with crowns and fixed dental prostheses or, in very advanced damage, with removable dentures.[165–167] Improved resin composite materials and adhesive systems make it possible to treat erosively damaged dentition much less invasively. Recently, the resistance of resin composite materials to abrasion has been much improved[140] and direct resin composite restorations show excellent longevity even under major stress.[141,168] Several case studies feature successful restoration of erosively and abrasively damaged dentition with the use of adhesive techniques.[169–172]

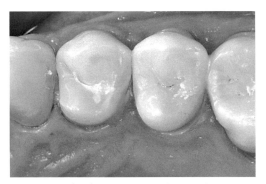

Fig 7-2   Occlusal erosions on teeth 24 and 25.

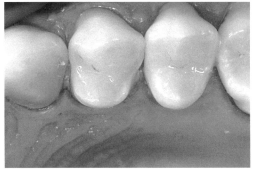

Fig 7-3   Sealing of occlusal erosions on teeth 24 and 25.

Fundamental principles of treating erosion:
1. Determine and eliminate the cause(s) of substance loss, a prerequisite for longevity of restorative and reconstructive measures
2. Preventive, restorative, and reconstructive measures, which are determined by the severity of substance loss (eg, loss of vertical dimension); treatment is minimally invasive
3. Adequate follow-up examinations and professional maintenance of reconstructions.

Sealing

In order to prevent functional and esthetic problems, teeth with erosive and abrasive damage should be treated even in their initial stages. The minimally invasive treatment is sealing of the damaged tooth surface (Figs 7-2 and 7-3).

Clinical experience shows that sealing diminishes hypersensitivity; however, it has to be repeated every 6 to 9 months.[173]

Direct resin composite restorations

Occlusal erosions typically present with indentations on crown cusps, as well as overlapping fillings. These defects can reach the dentin and maintain a decrease in pH for longer after acid exposure (unpublished data). To prevent further progression of erosive lesions, affected areas should be treated locally with direct resin composite restorations (Figs 7-4 and 7-5). Composite is considered superior to conventional glass-ionomer cement as filling material as the latter can disintegrate in acidic environments.[174] Direct resin composite restorations are the treatment of choice if the surrounding tooth substance is healthy or provided with satisfactory fillings. The treatment can be considered a minimally invasive strategy.

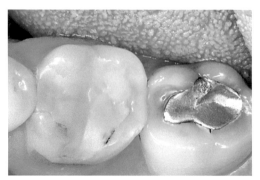

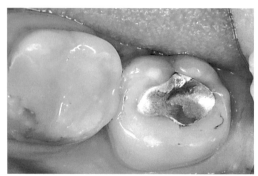

Fig 7-4 *Occlusal erosion on tooth 37. The edges of amalgam filling are rising above the level of adjacent tooth surfaces.*

Fig 7-5 *The erosively damaged parts on tooth 37 were filled with resin composite as a minimally invasive treatment.*

Composite and ceramic reconstructions

As long as intraocclusal loss of tooth substance is minimal and the anatomical shape persists, teeth can be restored directly with resin composite materials. The increase in the vertical dimension is frequently minimal and easily accepted by the patient. Teeth may be directly reconstructed by the practitioner without needing further means of support for a tooth, according to its original anatomy or with a splint technique.[172] This technique can be used not only with occlusal lesions, but also to restore other local (eg, vestibular or oral) defects (Case reports 3 and 4). The advantage of this method is the defect-focused approach, which protects the remaining tooth substance.

More difficult situations arise when there is severe substance loss and loss of the original anatomy. Substance loss is frequently extensive vertically as well as vestibularly–orally, necessitating full ceramic reconstructions. Patients often present only when changes in (maxillary) incisors become visible. A frequent reason to seek treatment is crumbling and transparent incisor edges. For esthetic as well as functional reasons, treatment with veneers or veneer crowns is indicated for extensive anterior erosions (Case report 8). Lateral teeth presenting with extended defects on two or more surfaces, including large vertical substance loss, might indicate treatment with resin composite or full ceramic overlays (Case reports 5, 6, 8, and 9). This strategy enables esthetic and functional rehabilitation with maximal protection of tooth substance. It has to be noted that these reconstructions are complex and expensive, and that longevity can be guaranteed only with accompanying preventive measures. Regular follow-ups are vital.

With heavily damaged teeth where there is a substantial vertical dimension affected, the anatomy and functionality have to be extensively reconstructed.

In these cases, ceramic crowns and fixed dental prostheses are indicated, and the degree of destruction of each individual tooth will determine the specific combination of restoration techniques utilized. Adhesive techniques are to be preferred because of the excellent acid resistance of resin composite adhesives (as discussed above). In every case and for every tooth, the most minimally invasive method should be chosen.

Choice of reconstructive method and restoration material:

Tooth substance loss

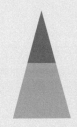

Restoration

Sealing

Direct composite restoration

Composite reconstruction

Ceramic reconstruction

Ceramic crown and fixed dental prosthesis/

removable denture

■ = no loss of vertical dimension
■ = loss of vertical dimension

The method of restoration and the choice of material depend on the degree of destruction of the tooth. For every individual tooth, the most minimally invasive method should be chosen!

Case reports

Case report 1 (Figs 7-6 to 7-16)

Direct resin composite restorations in combination with orthodontic therapy

Carola Imfeld, Preventive Dentistry and Oral Epidemiology, University of Zurich

Diagnosis: erosions in teeth 13 to 23 orally as well as teeth 14 and 24 occlusally and orally.
Restorations: pulp protection with resin composite on teeth 12 to 22; orthodontic treatment; long-term provisional solution with resin composite reconstructions in teeth 13 to 23.

Description

The 20-year-old woman initially presented with advanced stage defects of dental hard tissue in maxillary anterior teeth accompanied by hypersensitivity and compromised appearance. General history had no distinctive features apart from the consumption of approximately 10 cigarettes per day. One specific feature with respect to the possible involvement of stomach acid was that she had suffered from strong weekly migraine attacks that induced regular vomiting, not followed by mechanical oral hygiene, until the age of 14 years. Despite there being no direct indications for gastroesophageal reflux, examination by a gastroenterologist was initiated. Apart from a small axial hiatus hernia, severe gastroesophageal reflux could be excluded. To prevent further loss of dental hard tissue, prophylactic medication was considered. In order to exclude dietary factors, a detailed questionnaire was filled out, without showing significant results. There were no signs of reduced salivary flow rate and parafunctions. Oral hygiene was unsatisfactory and periodontal examination showed generalized gingivitis.

Diagnosis

Advanced stage localized erosions of endogenous nature, probably resulting from regular vomiting. Subsequent elongation of the anterior teeth in the maxilla, requiring general orthodontic treatment.

Therapy

Because of the elongation of the anterior teeth until occlusal contact, there was no space for oral restoration of the maxillary anterior teeth. No loss of the vertical dimension had occurred as the lateral teeth were not affected, or only minimally affected, by erosion. Orthodontic treatment was indicated independent of the erosive damage, which then provided the necessary space for oral treatment of the maxillary anterior teeth. Teeth 12 to 22 were orally restored with resin composite to protect the pulp. As a long-term solution, full ceramic crowns were planned for teeth 11 and 21, and direct resin composite reconstructions for teeth 13, 12, 22, and 23. Orthodontic measures were taken to enable correct anatomical reconstruction. Removal of the two maxillary premolars damaged by erosion, 14 and 24, was necessary for orthodontic reasons. At intervals, a further resin composite layer was applied orally to teeth 12 to 22. All teeth were examined bi-annually for erosion progression. No new erosions were discovered, making further gastroenterological measures unnecessary. Immediately after debonding, the teeth were reconstructed anatomically correct with resin composite using rubber dam technique, acid etching, and total bonding. The patient was happy with the resin composite solutions, to the point of deciding to postpone ceramic crown work to a later stage. After completion, the patient did not appear for her yearly dental hygenist's appointments. Other than local polishing of the resin composite and replacement of a filling in tooth 27, no other maintenance was necessary.

Discussion

The young woman presented with no or minimal erosive involvement of lateral teeth. There were no caries lesions and only sparse occlusal fillings. Orthodontic intervention was indicated to reach a correct occlusion and to simultaneously provide space for restorative measures in the maxillary anterior teeth. Healthy dental hard tissue of the minimally affected lateral teeth could be protected. This treatment strategy, however, implies the patient's willingness to wear an orthodontic device over an extended period of time. As the resin composite reconstructions were not planned as a long-term solution, individual characteristics and coloring were not considered. The patient was, however, happy with the appearance even after 4 years and it was, therefore, decided to keep the reconstructions as a long-term provisional solution.

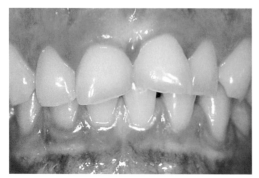

Fig 7-6   Initial frontal view with loss of incisal edges.

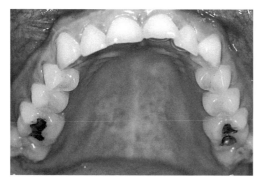

Fig 7-7   Initial view of maxillary teeth with erosions.

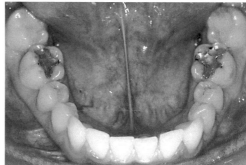

Fig 7-8   Initial view of the mandible.

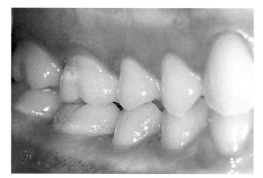

Fig 7-9   Initial right lateral view.

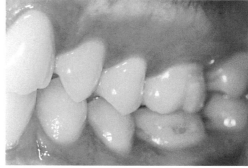

Fig 7-10   Initial left lateral view.

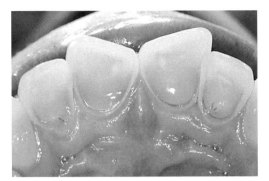

Fig 7-11 *Initial detailed view of anterior maxilla orally, featuring advanced erosions.*

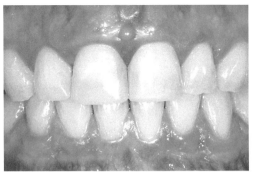

Fig 7-12 *Frontal view after orthodontic treatment and 4 years after restoration of teeth 13 to 23 with direct resin composite reconstructions before polishing.*

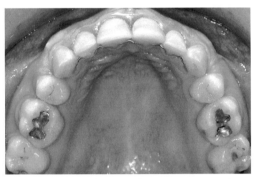

Fig 7-13 *Maxilla after orthodontic treatment and 4 years after restoration of teeth 13 to 23 with direct resin composite before polishing.*

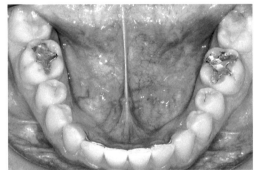

Fig 7-14 *Mandible after orthodontic treatment before polishing.*

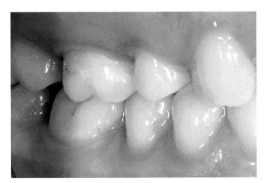

Fig 7-15 *Right lateral view after orthodontic treatment and 4 years after restoration of teeth 13 to 23 with direct resin composite before polishing.*

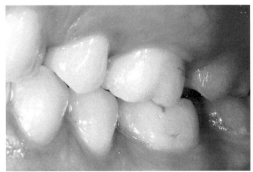

Fig 7-16 *Left lateral view after orthodontic treatment and 4 years after restoration of teeth 13 to 23 with direct resin composite before polishing.*

Case report 2 (Figs 7-17 to 7-28)

Direct resin composite restorations

Nadine Schlueter, Conservative and Preventive Dentistry, Justus-Liebig University, Giessen

Diagnosis: generalized erosions on occlusal and oral tooth surfaces.
Restorations: direct resin composite restorations without increase in vertical dimension.

Description

A 34-year-old man presented with distinct defects on occlusal surfaces as well as on oral surfaces of the maxillary incisors and canines. General medical history was without pathological findings. The specific workup included a nutrition recording over a period of 1 week, which showed frequent consumption of a soft drink containing phosphoric acid and a vegetarian diet with an increased fruit and juice consumption. The acidic beverages were sipped throughout the day; in addition the patient rinsed with the soft drink. Defects were found on occlusal surfaces of the molars and premolars in the maxilla and the mandible, resulting in a loss of the occlusal relief, as well as of dental hard tissue on the oral surfaces of the maxillary incisors. The gingival and periodontal conditions and the mucosa were normal. The oral hygiene was good; plaque was found only on isolated areas.

Diagnosis

Generalized erosions caused by exogenous factors on oral and occlusal tooth surfaces, requiring no therapeutic measures with regard to the vertical dimension. Isolated caries, class III malocclusion with one-sided cross-bite.

Therapy

Reduction of acid intake and the use of a fluoride-containing mouthrinse were recommended in order to prevent further dental substance loss through acid exposure. Additionally, general recommendations with respect to oral hygiene were given. After the stabilization of the oral situation, the defects were directly restored with resin composite without further loss of healthy dental hard tissue in the preparation measures. Any fillings that were inadequate were removed and the defects were integrated into the restorations. For the restoration of molars and premolars, a micro-hybrid resin composite was used with incremental technique. First, the mandibular molars were restored, taking into account the construction of a compensatory curve. An increase in vertical dimension was avoided. Second, the maxillary molars were reconstructed quadrant by quadrant. As soon as sufficient occlusal support was achieved in the molars, the premolars were reconstructed in a similar manner. For incisors and canines, an ultrafine particle hybrid resin composite was used as it has superior coloring and polishing properties. Oral surfaces of teeth 13, 12, 22, and 23 were overlayed. Additionally, the incisal edges of teeth 12, 11, 21, and 22 were reconstructed.

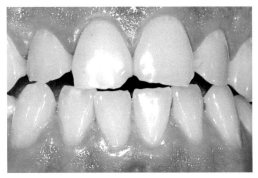

Fig 7-17   *Vestibular view of teeth 3 to 3 in occlusion before treatment.*

Discussion

Covering erosive defects without progression tendencies with resin composite is a minimally invasive treatment strategy. The remaining tooth substance of patients with erosions is often free of caries and fillings. In addition, where there is remaining vertical dimension, space is often scarce, and preparations for laboratory-fabricated restorations such as crowns or overlays require further loss of healthy tooth substance.

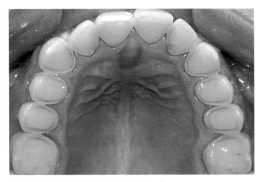

Fig 7-18   *Initial view of the maxilla.*

Regular follow-up examinations for this patient show a stabilized situation over the last 5 years. Neither loss of restorations nor discolorations was observed. Regular bitewing imaging of approximal spaces indicated no marginal leakage or approximal caries.

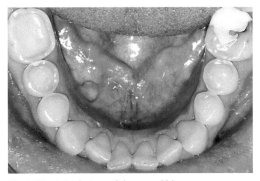

Fig 7-19   *Initial view of the mandible.*

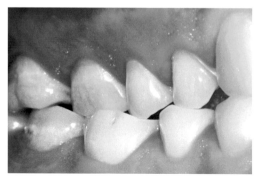

Fig 7-20 *Initial view in occlusion of the 1st and 4th quadrants.*

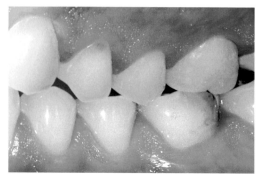

Fig 7-21 *Initial view in occlusion of the 2nd and 3rd quadrants.*

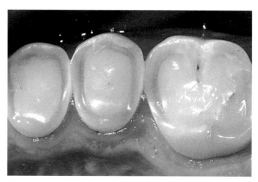

Fig 7-22 *Detailed view of the lesions on teeth 24 to 26.*

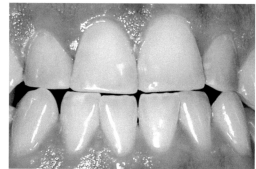

Fig 7-23 *Vestibular view after reconstruction of teeth 3 to 3 in occlusion.*

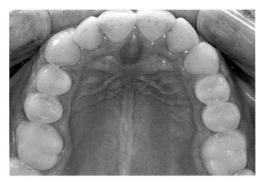

Fig 7-24   *Maxilla after reconstruction.*

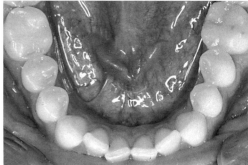

Fig 7-25   *Mandible after reconstruction.*

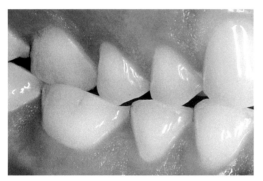

Fig 7-26   *View in occlusion of 1st and 4th quadrants after reconstruction.*

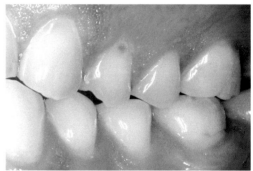

Fig 7-27   *View in occlusion of 2nd and 3rd quadrants after reconstruction.*

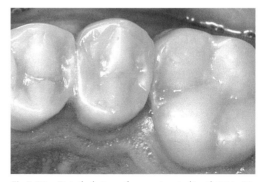

Fig 7-28   *Detailed view of reconstructed teeth 24 to 26.*

Case report 3 (Figs 7-29 to 7-42)

Composite reconstructions with a splint technique

Patrick R. Schmidlin, Olivier O. Schicht, and Thomas Attin, Clinic for Preventive Dentistry, Periodontology and Cariology, University of Zurich

Reconstructing substance loss traditionally has required crowns for the affected areas.[175] This heavily invasive treatment meant large additional loss of healthy tooth substance. Improved adhesive systems make substance-friendly treatment possible, such as use of ceramic occlusal overlays in lateral dentition.[171] Nevertheless, applying these externally constructed devices still requires the loss of some additional tooth substance during preparation. Direct restoration with resin composite seems to be done only rarely at present for extensive oral reconstructive treatment of erosive substance damage. However, the advantages include both the minimally invasive nature of the treatment and also its relatively low costs.

We have developed a technique to replace lost tooth substance with the use of an occlusal splint technique with direct adhesive resin composite restoration occlusally.[172,176] A case control study showed that stable results could be observed 3 years after the reconstruction.[177] The following section describes the technique and illustrates the clinical treatment with a cast (Case report 3); this is followed by a current case report (Case report 4).

Pretreatment/treatment planning

After careful clinical examination, casts of the mandible and maxilla as well as the facebow and/or bite registration are produced. A detailed analysis of the mounted casts provides the basis for the treatment plan, including considerations of the vertical dimension and the individual situation in the jaws. Alternative strategies are available if treatment is required in both jaws. One approach is to reconstruct the teeth in one jaw with the use of the occlusal splint technique, with the other jaw subsequently being restored with external reconstructions or also with the occlusal splint technique. Another strategy, indicated specifically if one row of teeth shows only minor substance loss, is direct resin composite reconstruction on the jaw. Subsequently, after making a fresh cast of the reconstructed jaw, a cast of the other jaw is made to allow dental articulation to be assessed before the teeth in the other jaw are reconstructed with the use of occlusal splint technique. Depending on the desired increase in the vertical dimension, it can be useful to prepare the patient for the altered situation and to prevent any joint conditions developing by building a stabilizing splint before clinical reconstruction.[178,179] Once the treatment plan has been made and all the materials and papers are in place, dental technicians can fix the desired vertical dimension in the articulator and provide a waxup of the selected lateral dentition areas. The waxup excludes the outermost anterior and distal lateral teeth of every quadrant, unless sufficient support for the splint is provided by buccal, labial, or oral tooth surfaces. Finally, the wax-up cast has to be doubled and the splint formed on the plaster.

Clinical procedure

The procedure is described here for an example case involving teeth 4–7. After any local anesthesia has been administered, the teeth are dried with a rubber-dam technique and cleaned with polishing paste. The teeth can be separated with transparent plastic or steel matrix bands, or with teflon foil, which should be inserted carefully, if necessary with the help of a spatula. Before and after separation, the stability and fit of the splint should be ensured. The goal is for the splint to make visible the lost tooth substance as modeled in the waxup. It might be necessary to modify the splint, particularly in the area of the distal rubberdam retainer. Subsequently, teeth 4 and 6 are prepared for adhesion. Preparatory measures depend on the adhesion and resin composite system chosen for the treatment. We recommend mechanical roughening with an airborne-particle abrasion instrument (aluminum oxide powder) and etching of enamel with phosphoric acid for at least 30 seconds. Remains of resin composite fillings that are considered relevant clinically and radiologically should be covered with silane. It can be useful to replace older extensive fillings before occlusal restoration. Smaller fillings can

be applied during the occlusal splint technique. Subsequently, further conditioning steps are taken and the adhesive applied. The amount of resin composite required to replace the missing tooth substance is applied to the teeth and splint, the latter then being positioned slowly with moderate pressure. Excess material is removed before light curing. Photopolymerization is performed for 3 to 4 seconds to achieve a superficial hardening of the resin composite. The splint is carefully removed. Remaining overlaps are then cut with the scalpel. In the next step, final photopolymerization is carried out occlusally, bucally, and orally for 60 seconds each. After rough finishing of the first reconstructed tooth, particularly interdentally, tooth 5 is then equally treated. Reconstructing tooth 7 is finally done directly or with the help of the splint. When both quadrants of one jaw have been restored, precision adjustment of occlusion is performed. The treatment is concluded with polishing of the restorations.

Discussion

The use of resin composite in reconstructions of lateral teeth, while still being somewhat controversial in the literature, is regularly done clinically.[141,180] Nevertheless, resin composite is still used conservatively in extensive direct reconstruction because of the high wearing rates that might occur and uncertainty over the long-term prognosis. Furthermore, the technique can demanding in terms of technical skill and time. *In vivo* studies have only presented approximate results and recommendations with respect to wearing rates, and long-term prognosis is difficult to make because of the large variations of filling materials used.[108,147,181] The complex process described above has, however, shown good results in our clinic. The experience in the last 3 years has been positive and acceptance with patients is high.[177]

As a rule, the long-term prognosis of direct resin composite reconstructions relies not only on the materials used but also on clinical planning, application skills of the dentist, lifestyle of the patient, and oral hygiene.[168] The treatment method presented here is only one of many options. Nevertheless, factors like cost–benefit ratio and minimal invasiveness are valid advantages of this method for the private practice.

Step-by-step procedure

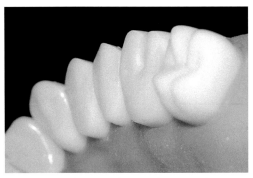

Fig 7-29 Initial view of the irregular occlusal erosive defects in lateral teeth (simulation on a cast).

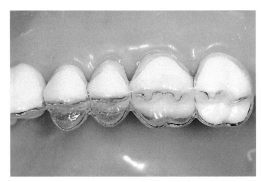

Fig 7-30 In situ splint extending to the gingiva edge. The fit should be without stress. The hollow space created by the waxup where tooth substance is to be replaced is visible.

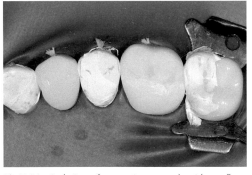

Fig 7-31 Isolation of approximate teeth with a teflon strip.

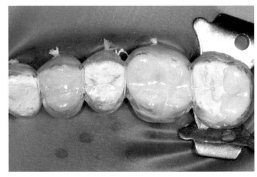

Fig 7-32 Insertion of a support device for the isolated teeth.

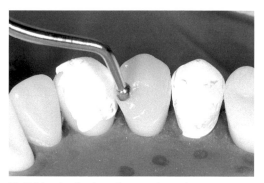

Fig 7-33 *Application of restorative resin composite on the prepared tooth surface.*

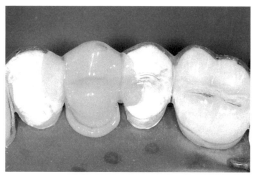

Fig 7-34 *Fitted splint filled with resin composite. Overlaps can easily be removed before initial primary photopolymerization.*

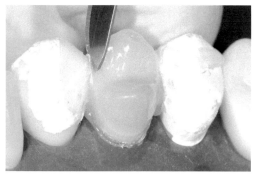

Fig 7-35 *After initial primary polymerization for 3 seconds, the splint is carefully stripped and remaining overlaps removed with the scalpel before final photopolymerization.*

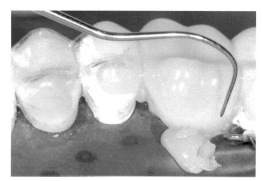

Fig 7-36 *Identical procedure in the next tooth in the quadrant.*

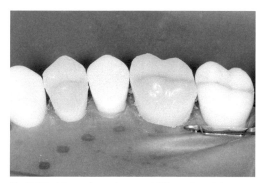

Fig 7-37 *View of rough cast of fillings. Special attention should be paid to approximal surfaces to enable final polishing between restorations.*

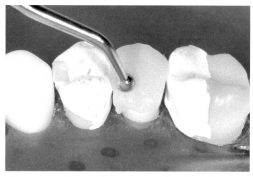

Fig 7-38 *Isolation of reconstructed teeth with teflon foil and application of resin composite to the tooth being treated.*

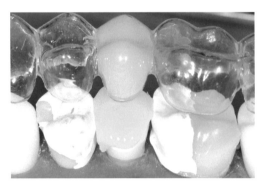

Fig 7-39   Splint filled with resin composite before fitting.

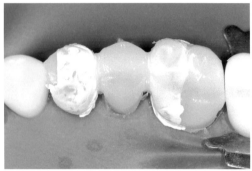

Fig 7-40   View of the quadrant after stripping away the splint and before definite polymerization.

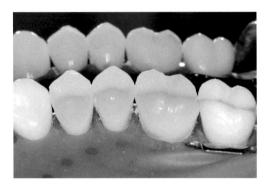

Fig 7-41   View after rough casting.

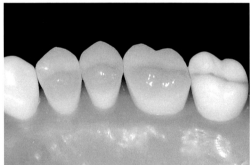

Fig 7-42   Complete and polished resin composite reconstructions after rubberdam removal.

Case report 4 (Figs 7-43 to 7-56)

Reconstructions with direct resin composite splint technique and ceramic crowns

Oliver O. Schicht, Preventive Dentistry and Oral Epidemiology, University of Zurich

Diagnosis: multiple dental erosions on occlusal, vestibular, and oral tooth surfaces.

Restorations: increase in vertical dimension by >2 mm with direct resin composite reconstructions with the use of a splint technique; full ceramic crowns on teeth 13 to 23.

Description

A 24-year-old woman was referred by a center for eating disorders as she had visible dental defects. Bulimia as the underlying cause had remitted and the patient had not suffered a relapse for several months. The patient continued psychotherapy and a small daily dose of antidepressant. Other than regular smoking, the previous medical history was inconspicuous. During the specific workup, the patient admitted to not having seen a dental clinician for 20 years because of a fear of dentists. The patient had no symptoms from the teeth other than her esthetic problems. The subsequent examination revealed extensive erosions. Furthermore, amalgam fillings were insufficient and there were caries lesions in lateral teeth. Vitality testing with carbon dioxide showed positive results for all teeth. Minor attrition defects were also found on lateral teeth. Distinct parafunction was, however, not discernible. The appearance of the erosions confirmed current absence of erosive factors on tooth substance. Loss of vertical dimension was estimated at approximately 3 mm. There was no indication for decreased salivary flow rate. Periodontally, localized gingivitis and occasional recessions were observed.

Diagnosis

Generalized inactive endogenous erosions with loss of vertical dimension due to previous eating disorder, which remains actively treated; additional primary and secondary caries in lateral teeth.

Therapy

Minimally invasive reconstruction was used to achieve an increase in vertical dimension of 2–3 mm. Because this was a small increase, use of an occlusal splint seemed unnecessary. As the erosive defects were less distinct in the mandible than the maxilla, the mandibular lateral teeth, followed by the mandibular incisors, were directly reconstructed with resin composite, resulting in a vertical dimension increase of approximately 1 mm. Caries was treated simultaneously. Subsequently, the maxillary lateral teeth 14–16 and 24–26 were reconstructed with resin composite, using a splint based on a waxup produced by the dental technician. Teeth 17 and 27 were directly reconstructed with resin composite. As in the mandible, caries was treated simultaneously using the increment technique. The reconstruction of tooth morphology in the maxilla resulted in an additional increase in vertical dimension by approximately 1.5 mm and was immediately accepted by the patient. Because of her smoking habit and the need for esthetic durability, as well as the considerable loss of tooth substance, it was decided after long consultations with the patient to refrain from using resin composite reconstruction in the maxillary anterior teeth. Soon afterwards, therefore, the reconstruction of anterior teeth 13 to 23 was performed with full ceramic crowns, with a provisional solution provided by the dental technician. In order to enhance anterior esthetics, which was affected by both loss of tooth substance and an unfavorable gingival line, a labially restricted surgical crown lengthening of teeth 11 and 21 had been performed even before treatment was initiated. The result pleased the patient both functionally and esthetically.

Discussion

The chosen treatment aimed at replacing lost tooth substance. Composite was chosen because it can be applied without much preparation requiring further loss of tooth substance. The reconstruction with splint technique facilitated occlusal adaptations in connection with the increase in the vertical dimension. Although this technique requires large amounts of increment increase on the tooth, the morphological situation results in a relatively small C-factor, meaning that no relevant reduction of filling and border qualities are to be expected. With respect to longevity, it is favorable that the underlying cause no longer persists. Realistically, longevity has to be considered to be restricted by material properties. In addition, the patient's smoking habit is detrimental to the esthetic quality of the resin composite reconstructions. Nevertheless, because of the relatively young age of the patient, minimally invasive treatment seemed to be the right choice. Naturally, regular follow-up examinations should be performed.

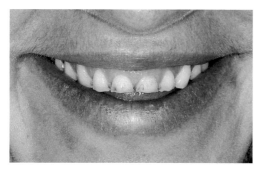

Fig 7-43 *Initial view of smiling patient. There is esthetically unpleasing gingival exposure because of the sloping gingiva line from tooth 3 to 1.*

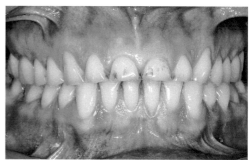

Fig 7-44 *Initial frontal view.*

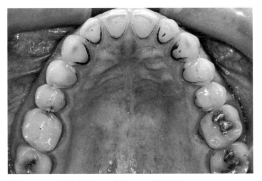

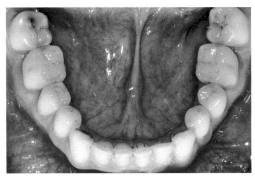

Fig 7-45 *Initial view of the maxilla. There are generalized distinct inactive erosions with extended dentin exposition, approximal caries in tooth 15 distally, occlusally in tooth 17, and recurrent caries in teeth 26 and 27.*

Fig 7-46 *Initial view of the mandible. There is inactive occlusal and buccal erosions and occlusal caries in tooth 47.*

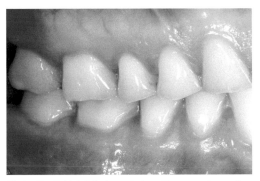

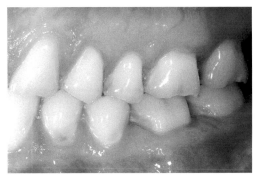

Fig 7-47 *Initial right lateral view. Decrease in tooth morphology with loss of vertical dimension.*

Fig 7-48 *Initial left lateral view. Decrease in tooth morphology with loss of vertical dimension.*

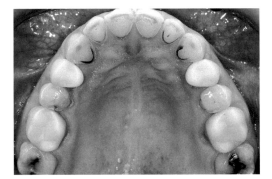

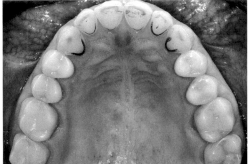

Fig 7-49 *View after reconstruction of teeth 14, 24, 16, and 26. Insufficient amalgam filling in tooth 26 was replaced with resin composite during the reconstruction of the occlusal surface.*

Fig 7-50 *View after complete reconstruction of the maxillary lateral teeth. The caries lesion in tooth 15 distally was treated with an increment hardening technique during reconstruction of the occlusal surface with splint technique. Teeth 17 and 27 were restored directly with resin composite after caries removal.*

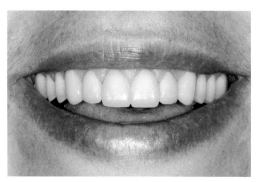

Fig 7-51 *View of smiling patient after completed treatment. Gingiva exposure on central incisors could be diminished, gingiva line appears more pleasing.*

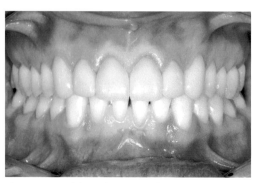

Fig 7-52 *Final frontal view. Teeth 13 to 23 were treated with full ceramic crowns.*

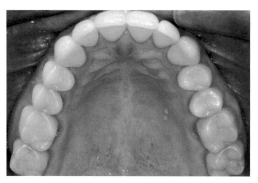

Fig 7-53 *View of the maxilla after completion of the reconstruction.*

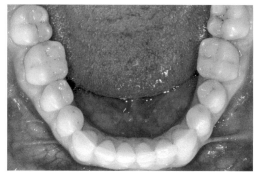

Fig 7-54 *View of the mandible after completion of the reconstruction. Laterally, there was only occasionally large tooth substance losses occlusally and buccally and these were directly restored with resin composite. Occlusal caries on tooth 47 was treated at this time.*

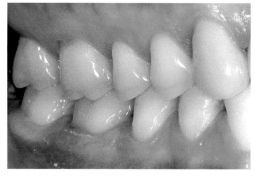

Fig 7-55 *Right lateral view after completion of the reconstruction.*

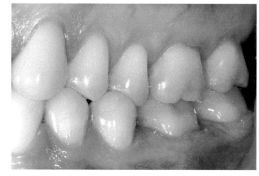

Fig 7-56 *Left lateral view after completion of the reconstruction.*

Case report 5 (Figs 7-57 to 7-71)

Direct resin composite restorations and indirect resin composite overlays
Carola Imfeld, Preventive Dentistry and Oral Epidemiology, University of Zurich

Diagnosis: multiple dental erosions on buccal, occlusal, and oral tooth surfaces, partly combined with attrition.
Restorations: increase in vertical dimension by >2 mm with direct resin composite reconstructions and indirect resin composite overlays in lateral teeth; therapy of remaining defects with direct resin composite restorations.

Description
A clinician had proposed that a 31-year-old man should have full crown restorations on at least his premolar and molar teeth, including clinical crown lengthening procedure to treat the defects in dental hard tissue. Frightened by the invasiveness of the therapy and of the high costs, the patient inquired about alternative therapies and was then referred to our clinic. General medical history was inconspicuous. The specific case history revealed painful dentin hypersensitivity upon taking acidic beverages and food that had been ongoing for several years. Radiographic records showed that the major part of the loss of dental hard tissue had taken place over a period of approximately 2 years that occurred 10–8 years prior to the present examination. Only

slight deterioration had occurred since that time. Specific questioning with respect to reflux-related symptoms (also in the past) proved negative. A written and oral workup of dietary habits was inconspicuous. Advanced stage erosive defects were found on all occlusal surfaces of lateral teeth, as well as palatally on maxillary incisors and localized on buccal surfaces. Attrition was also apparent. The patient confirmed bruxism. Periodontal examination was without pathological findings and salivary flow rate proved physiological.

Diagnosis
Advanced stage, inactive, idiopathic erosions, combined with symptoms of attrition and abrasion.

Therapy
After being presented with various therapeutic options, the patient decided for direct resin composite reconstruction of the maxilla as well as of teeth 34 to 44 and 47. For the teeth 37, 36, 35, 45, and 46, resin composite overlays were planned. Wisdom teeth were to be extracted. In a first step, the maxillary lateral teeth were directly reconstructed and the vertical dimension increased. In a second step, resin composite overlays were inserted in the above-mentioned teeth of the mandible. The dental technician adapted the occlusion to the direct reconstructions in the maxilla and identified necessary corrections. The vertical dimension was thereby further increased. Teeth 34, 44, and

47, which were only slightly affected by erosion, were directly reconstructed with resin composite. As a result of the restoration of the vertical dimension, there was enough space to restore the anterior teeth with resin composite. Buccal erosions were treated in the same way. All adhesive restorations were performed using rubberdam, etching technique, and total bonding. In a follow-up examination, teeth were polished and a Michigan-splint for the maxilla was made.

The patient returned for yearly follow-up examinations, including dental hygiene. During maintenance, local polishing of the resin composite, repair of a chipping in tooth 23, and reinsertion of a loosened overlay on tooth 35 became necessary. Worn-out areas as well as a fracture in the Michigan-splint had to be repaired.

Discussion

The erosive lesions of the teeth could be restored in a manner that was both minimally invasive and cost effective, according to the patient's wishes. Maintenance of the restorations involved only minor repairs. After 7 years, the resin composite displays visible wear, particularly in the maxillary lateral teeth. Nevertheless, the presented therapy is considered advantageous, particularly in younger patients, for its protection of healthy dental hard tissue and long-term preservation of dental health. Given the fact that the resin composite overlays proved more wear resistant than the direct resin composite reconstructions, one might consider also using indirect resin composite restorations in the antagonistic positions to overlays. Ceramic reconstructions would probably have been more stable over the described period of time. However, they would have required more invasive preparatory measures and might have fractured during the patient's ongoing bruxism. The patient reported that he would again choose the presented therapy, despite inferior wear resistance and esthetic appearance of the resin composite compared with a ceramic solution.

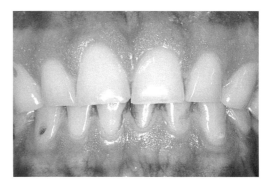

Fig 7-57   *Initial frontal view with labial erosions.*

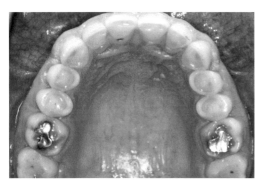

Fig 7-58   *Initial view of the maxilla, with erosions and signs of attrition.*

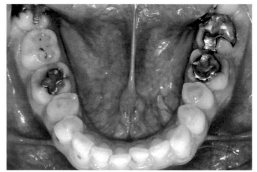

Fig 7-59   *Initial view of the mandible, with erosions and signs of attrition.*

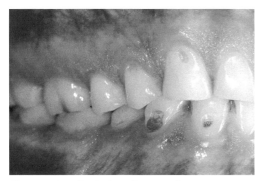

Fig 7-60   *Initial right lateral view with erosions.*

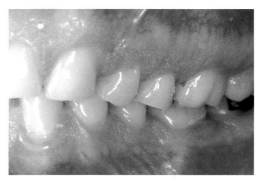

Fig 7-61   *Initial left lateral view with erosions.*

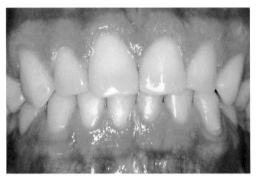

Fig 7-62 *Frontal view after direct resin composite reconstruction.*

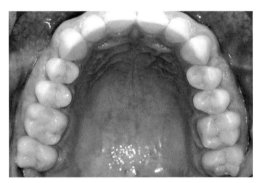

Fig 7-63 *Maxilla after direct resin composite reconstruction.*

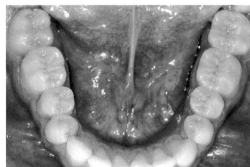

Fig 7-64 *Mandible with resin composite overlays in teeth 37 to 35, 45, and 46, as well as direct resin composite reconstructions in teeth 34 to 44 and 47.*

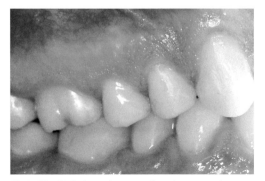

Fig 7-65 *Right lateral view with resin composite overlays in teeth 45 and 46 as well as direct resin composite reconstructions in the remaining teeth.*

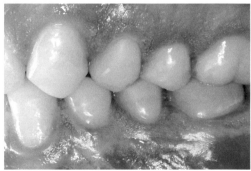

Fig 7-66 *Left lateral view with resin composite overlays in teeth 37 to 35 as well as direct resin composite reconstructions in the remaining teeth.*

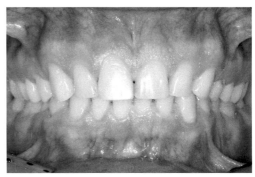

Fig 7-67 *Frontal view without prior polishing, 7 years after reconstructive therapy.*

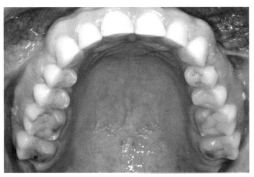

Fig 7-68 *Maxilla without prior polishing, 7 years after reconstructive therapy.*

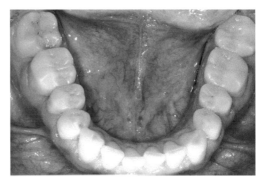

Fig 7-69 *Mandible without prior polishing, 7 years after reconstructive therapy.*

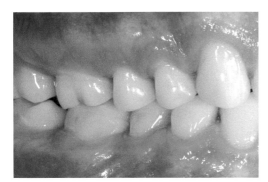

Fig 7-70 *Right side without prior polishing, 7 years after reconstructive therapy.*

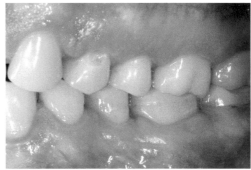

Fig 7-71 *Left side without prior polishing, 7 years after reconstructive therapy, showing loss of cervical filling in tooth 24.*

Case report 6 (Figs 7-72 to 7-91)

Indirect resin composite overlays and direct resin composite reconstructions

Nadine Schlueter, Conservative and Preventive Dentistry, Justus-Liebig University Giessen

Dental technician U. Tischler, Tischler Dental, Giessen

Diagnosis: generalized erosions on all tooth surfaces.

Restorations: increase in vertical dimension by 3 mm using a splint; restoration of the molars and premolars with laboratory-fabricated resin composite overlays; direct restoration of remaining defects with resin composite.

Description

A 20-year-old man with a general medical history without pathological findings had heavy consumption of sports and soft drinks, up to eight times a day, in addition to regular consumption of magnesium effervescent tablets in water (pH 4.7). He reported tooth sensitivity to temperature. Generalized non-carious caused defects on the vestibular, oral, and occlusal surfaces were visible. The severe loss of substance resulted in a decrease in the vertical dimension by approximately 3 mm. Occlusal support only remained on the third molar, the buccal cusp of tooth 16, and the canines. All other teeth showed no occlusion. A class III dysgnathia with crossbite on both sides and progenia in the

anterior mouth was found. The gingival and periodontal conditions were normal. Dental hygiene was good apart from the occasional occurrence of plaque. The remaining dentition was nearly completely unaffected by caries.

Diagnosis

Generalized erosions caused by exogenous factors resulting in a loss of vertical dimension of approximately 3 mm, combined with class III dysgnathia and cross-bite on both sides.

Therapy

Treatment was initiated with a nutritional consultation, where the patient was advised to replace sports and soft drinks with mineral water and the effervescent tablets with pills. It was recommended to use a stannous fluoride-containing mouthrinse with an acidic pH, which has proven most effective in the therapy of non-caries caused dental substance losses.[182] After stabilizing the dental situation, the reconstructive therapy was initiated. First, the vertical dimension was increased by approximately 3 mm with a splint. For 5 months, the splint was worn daily, if possible 24 hours a day, except during meals, dental hygiene, and sportive activity. At the beginning, the fit of the splint was monitored every other week, and later every 4 weeks. For the definite treatment of molars and premolars with resin composite overlays, the increase in vertical dimension was transferred to an articulator using the splint. The resin composite overlays were inserted under complete isolation using rubber-dam with an adhesive and flowable resin composite. Both jaws were subsequently restored in a single appointment each. In a next step, occlusion as well as laterotrusion, protrusion, and mediotrusion were carefully checked and adjusted where necessary. For the incisors of the maxilla, a waxup was made at the cast and a silicone matrix was made from this waxup. The maxillary incisors were subsequently reconstructed using an ultrafine-particle hybrid resin composite. In a last session, the edges of the mandibular incisors and canines were restored.

Discussion

Particularly in young patients, the treatment of severe erosive defects with loss of vertical dimension is often difficult. In most cases, reconstruction of all teeth using ceramic or ceramic-coated crowns is recommended; however, this requires large additional loss of tooth substance during the preparation measures. Such treatment also implies a large physical stress and is time and money consuming. Ceramic overlays require a smaller sacrifice with respect to tooth substance, but the financial aspect is equally demanding. Laboratory-fabricated resin composite overlays present a more cost-effective alternative. The new occlusion resulting from treatment with a splint can be directly transferred to the oral situation, showing better results both functionally and esthetically. Prior to definite restoration, it is of paramount importance to ensure proper dental hygiene and a stable dental situation with no progression of substance loss.

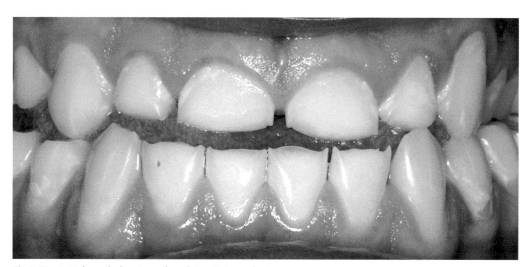

Fig 7-72 *Initial vestibular view of teeth 3 to 3 in occlusion.*

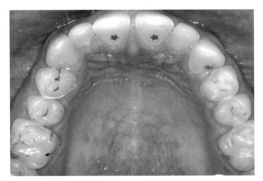

Fig 7-73 *Initial view of the maxilla; the stars are applied to measure erosion progression.*

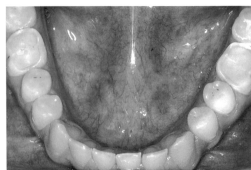

Fig 7-74 *Initial view of the mandible.*

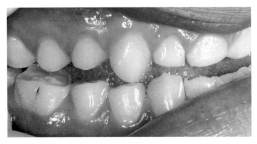

Fig 7-75 *Initial view of the 1st and 4th quadrants in occlusion.*

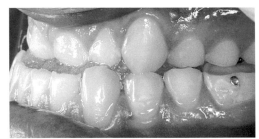

Fig 7-76 *Initial view of the 2nd and 3rd quadrants in occlusion.*

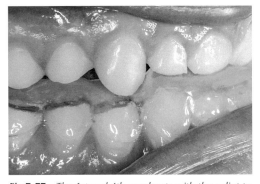

Fig 7-77 *The 1st and 4th quadrants with the splint to increase the vertical dimension.*

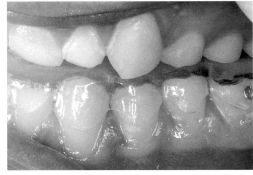

Fig 7-78 *The 2nd and 3rd quadrants with the splint to increase the vertical dimension.*

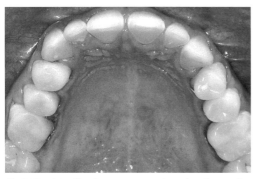

Fig 7-79   Maxilla after reconstruction of molars and premolars.

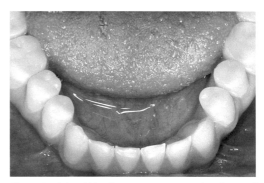

Fig 7-80   Mandible after reconstruction of molars and premolars.

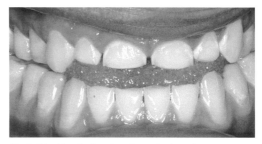

Fig 7-81   Vestibular view in occlusion after reconstruction of lateral teeth.

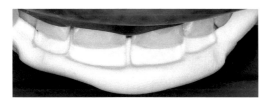

Fig 7-82   Fixed silicone matrix for reconstruction of maxillary incisors.

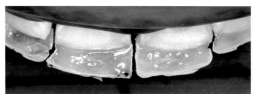

Fig 7-83   Imitation of oral enamel with flow resin composite.

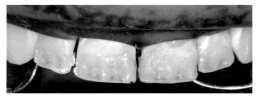

Fig 7-84   Layered application of an ultrafine-particle hybrid resin composite to imitate the body structure of the teeth.

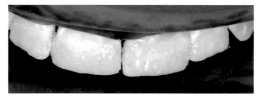

Fig 7-85   Reconstruction of vestibular enamel with an ultrafine-particle hybrid resin composite.

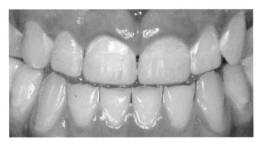

Fig 7-86   Vestibular view in occlusion after reconstruction of maxillary incisors and before reconstruction of mandibular incisors.

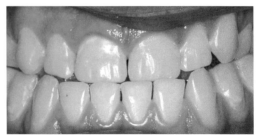

Fig 7-87   Vestibular view in occlusion after completed reconstruction.

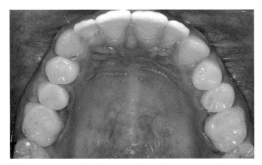

Fig 7-88   Maxilla after completed reconstruction.

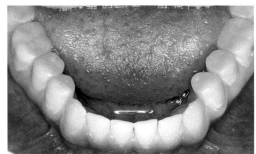

Fig 7-89   Mandible after completed reconstruction.

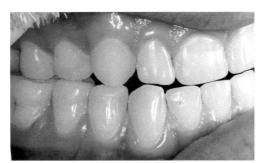

Fig 7-90   The 1st and 4th quadrants in occlusion after
completed reconstruction.

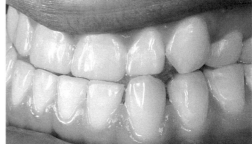

Fig 7-91   The 2nd and 3rd quadrants in occlusion
after completed reconstruction.

Case report 7 (Figs 7-92 to 7-109)

Direct resin composite restorations and crowns

Carola Imfeld, Preventive Dentistry and Oral Epidemiology, University of Zurich

Diagnosis: generalized erosions on oral and occlusal tooth surfaces.

Restorations: increase in vertical dimension by >2 mm following the Dahl principle and resin composite reconstructions; treatment of teeth 12 to 22 and 24 with porcelain-fused-to-metal (PFM) crowns and of the remaining defects with direct resin composite restorations.

Description

A 30-year-old man with advanced defects in dental hard tissue in the maxillary incisors required the most cost-effective treatment. General medical history had no specific features of relevance. The patient complained about increasing hypersensitivity in these teeth. A dietary history was unexceptional at the time, but the patient reported that he had consumed around 2 litres of cola daily, including deferred swallowing until some 3 years previously. Salivary flow rate was normal and there were no apparent parafunctions. Specific questioning with respect to reflux-related symptoms proved negative, but because of the obviously endogenous origin of the erosions (location), a gastroesophageal assessment was initiated, which revealed a gastroesophageal reflux condition. Respective conservative therapy and drug prescription was initiated. Teeth 21, 22, and 46 showed caries. Dental hygiene was unsatisfactory and periodontal examination revealed generalized gingivitis.

Diagnosis

Advanced endogenous erosions caused by gastroesophageal reflux, resulting in a loss of vertical dimension and elongation of anterior teeth; additional temporary dietary factors.

Therapy

Since the loss of dental hard tissue in the lateral teeth was much less pronounced than in maxillary anterior teeth, the patient was recommended to undergo orthodontic treatment to increase space, with subsequent restoration of the defects with direct resin composite and/or ceramic workpieces. As the patient was opposed to orthodontics and had limited financial resources, cheaper alternatives were offered. Despite being informed of the risks and the unpredictability of success, the patient opted for the application of the Dahl priniciple and direct resin composite restorations as a long-term provisional solution. In the meantime, tooth 12 had to be treated endodontically. In a first phase of treatment, teeth 13 to 23 were reconstructed twice (with 6-week interval) by adding resin composite material on the oral surfaces and increasing the vertical dimension by approximately 1.5 mm each time. Subsequently, the teeth were corrected to achieve good anterior occlusion. As a result, the lateral teeth remained without occlusal contacts and were left to elongation according to the Dahl principle. The patient accepted the increase in vertical dimension without symptoms and the lateral teeth exhibited elongation, which was, however, of varying extent and did not lead to occlusal contact in all teeth. After another 4 weeks, teeth 13 to 23 were again orally enlarged and the oral and/or occlusal surfaces of the maxillary lateral teeth were directly reconstructed with resin composite, apart from tooth 27. In a next step, the dental technician produced an occlusal waxup on casts of the mandibular lateral teeth, thereby adapting the occlusion to the resin composite reconstructions in the maxilla. A vacuum-formed splint was produced on the waxup. With the use of the splint, resin composite was applied occlusally to teeth 34 to 36 and 44 to 46. The mandibular anterior teeth as well as teeth 37 and 47 were directly restored with resin composite. In a last phase, PFM crowns were produced for teeth 12 to 22 and 24. Surgical harmonization of the gingiva line was not required by the patient. The patient appeared only irregularly for monitoring sessions and dental hygiene appointments. Other maintenance measures were not required. The last examination revealed damages in the resin composite reconstructions as

well as on the very thin ceramic oral layer of the PFM crowns, with visible metal on tooth 12. Tooth 47 showed filling margins projecting above the surrounding tooth surface. Upon questioning, the patient admitted to having ceased drug treatment of gastroesophageal reflux. The importance of the medical therapy was again explained to the patient.

Discussion

Despite the fact that the patient must have suffered from gastroesophageal reflux for several years, he was unaware of any symptoms. This common phenomenon is called silent reflux. General medical examination and therapy are of paramount importance. Because of the patient's rejection of orthodontic therapy, the Dahl principle was applied, which, however, allows no prediction with respect to tooth movement. In the present case, elongation only occurred partially. The remaining non-occlusion was compensated with direct resin composite reconstructions because of financial constraints. The gradually increasing thickness of the resin composite layer on the maxillary anterior teeth enabled the patient to achieve a slow adaptation; it was independent of his compliance and resulted in no functional or subjective problems. The patient ceased to treat his gastroesophageal reflux, which led to relapse and resulted in damaged reconstructions. After final elimination of all erosive factors, repair of the mandibular lateral reconstructions with direct resin composite or their replacement with indirect ceramic devices might be considered. The adjacent tooth substance would, however, remain prone to further erosion.

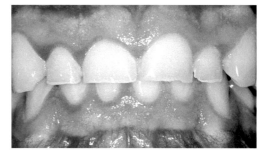

Fig 7-92   *Initial frontal view to show loss of edges on incisors and vertical dimension.*

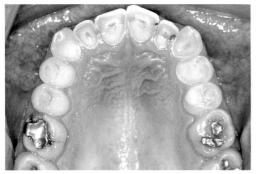

Fig 7-93   *Initial view of the maxilla showing generalized erosions.*

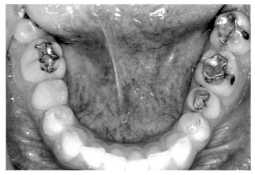

Fig 7-94   *Initial view of the mandible showing generalized erosions.*

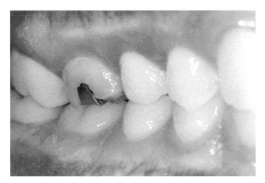

Fig 7-95   *Initial right lateral view showing decreased vertical dimension.*

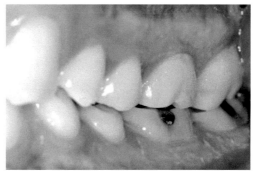

Fig 7-96   *Initial left lateral view with erosions and decreased vertical dimension.*

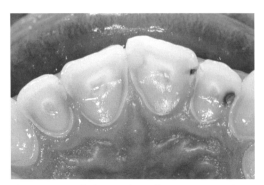

Fig 7-97 *Detailed view of maxillary anterior teeth orally with advanced stage of dental erosions and caries.*

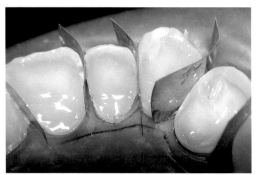

Fig 7-98 *Gradual reconstruction of oral erosions in teeth 13 to 23 by approximately 1.5 mm each time with direct resin composite.*

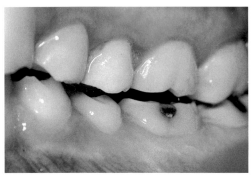

Fig 7-99 *Non-occlusion in lateral teeth as a result of the gradual direct resin composite reconstruction of teeth 13 to 23, following the Dahl principle.*

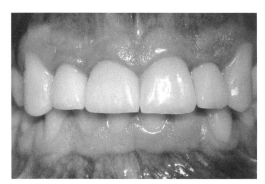

Fig 7-100 *Frontal teeth after PFM crowns in teeth 12 to 22 and direct resin composite reconstructions in teeth 13 and 23.*

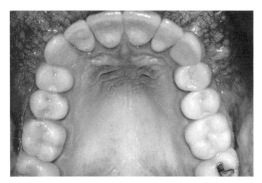

Fig 7-101 *Maxilla after PFM crowns in teeth 12 to 22 and 24 as well as direct resin composite reconstructions in all other teeth apart from tooth 27.*

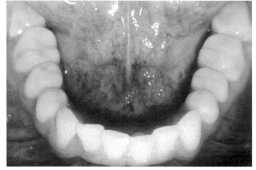

Fig 7-102 *Mandible after direct resin composite reconstruction with splint technique in teeth 36 to 34 and 44 to 46, as well as direct resin composite reconstructions in teeth 37, 33 to 43, and 47.*

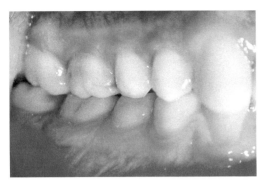

Fig 7-103   Right lateral view after direct resin composite reconstruction.

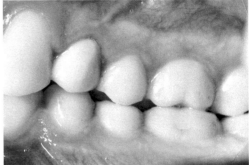

Fig 7-104   Left lateral view after direct resin composite reconstruction and PFM crown 24.

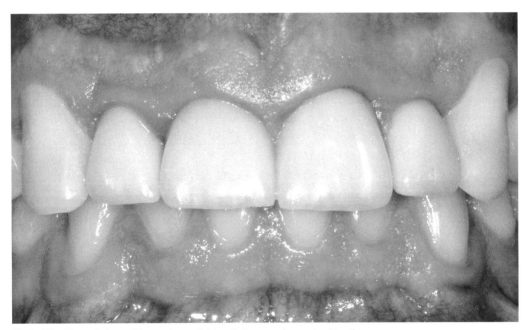

Fig 7-105   Frontal view without prior polishing, 3.5 years after restorative therapy.

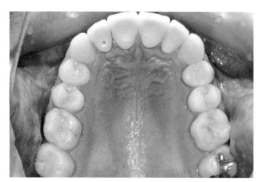

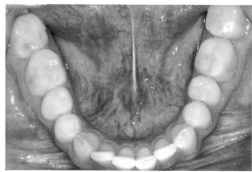

Fig 7-106 *Maxilla without prior polishing, 3.5 years after restorative therapy; the PFM crown 12 shows metal orally.*

Fig 7-107 *Mandible without prior polishing, 3.5 years after restorative therapy.*

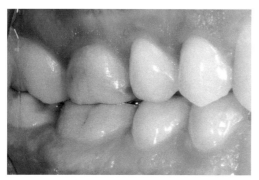

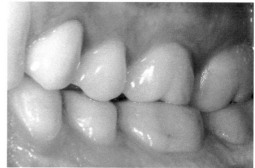

Fig 7-108 *Right lateral view without prior polishing, 3.5 years after restorative therapy.*

Fig 7-109 *Left lateral view without prior polishing, 3.5 years after restorative therapy.*

Case report 8
(Figs 7-110 to 7-124)

Direct resin composite restorations, ceramic overlays, and veneer crowns

Anne Grüninger, Department of Preventive, Restorative and Pediatric Dentistry, University of Bern

Diagnosis: multiple dental erosions on vestibular, occlusal, and oral tooth surfaces; angle class II with 12 mm overjet; loss of vertical dimension by approximately 2 mm.

Restorations: combined orthodontic and reconstructive therapy; treatment of erosions in lateral teeth with direct resin composite reconstructions, apart from teeth 16 and 46, which were provided with ceramic overlays; esthetic improvement of maxillary anterior teeth with veneer crowns.

Description

A 33-year-old woman was referred by the orthodontist for examination of erosions before therapy. A case history revealed that she used to be highly physically active both in endurance sports and in ski racing. Consumption of fruits and soft drinks was frequent. Caries control and erosion index investigation, radiography, and making of casts for modeling were completed prior to treatment. The patient was referred to a gastroenterologist because of suspected intrinsic factors causing erosion. Results with pH telemetry were negative and dietary habits also seemed unlikely as causes of the massive erosions; consequently, causes were not identified at that point. After orthodontic treatment, another history was obtained and at this point the patient admitted to having suffered from bulimia in the past. She was referred to a psychiatrist to assess her eating disorder. Partially remitted bulimia was diagnosed.

Diagnosis

Advanced stage of dental erosions with partially remitted bulimia; angle class II/1.

Therapy

After 16 months of orthodontic treatment, the following restorative therapy steps were initiated: (1) direct resin composite reconstructions in teeth 17, 15, 25 to 27, 37, 35, 33, 43 to 45, and 47; (2) ceramic overlays in teeth 16 and 46; (3) veneer crowns in teeth 13 to 23; and (4) resin composite reconstructions on vestibular surfaces of teeth 14 to 24.

Old fillings that were inadequate were replaced with resin composite and erosions were treated while reconstructing occlusion. Teeth 16 and 26 were then restored with ceramic overlays. Subsequently, teeth 13 to 23 were reconstructed with veneer crowns, conventionally prepared by the vestibular veneer design. Oral surfaces had lost so much substance that no preparation other than defining a clear border line was necessary. Teeth 14 to 24 then received vestibular resin composite reconstructions for esthetic reasons. During the first follow-up examination, the patient was again informed of preventive measures and was given a splint for fluoridization.

Discussion

Restorative therapy was unproblematic. The patient was highly motivated and applied prophylactic measures, which is of paramount importance for the durability of reconstructions. The esthetic result was considered optimal. Clinically, treatment proved stable after 2 years. The patient's dental hygiene continued to be very good.

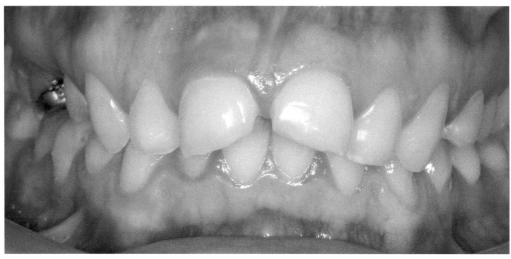

Fig 7-110   Initial vestibular view.

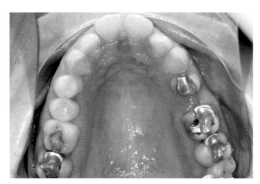

Fig 7-111   Initial occlusal view of the maxilla, with erosions in oral tooth surfaces 13 to 23 and severe proclination of incisors.

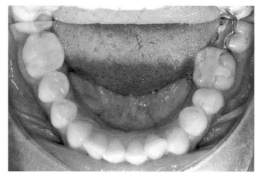

Fig 7-112   Initial occlusal view of the mandible, with erosions in occlusal surfaces in premolars.

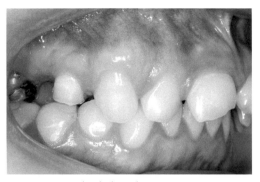

Fig 7-113   Initial right lateral view.

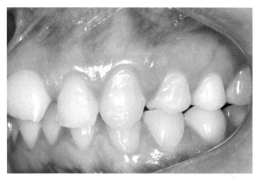

Fig 7-114   Initial left lateral view.

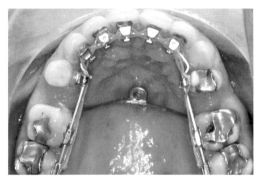

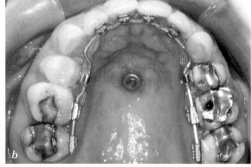

Fig 7-115a,b   Stages of orthodontic treatment in the maxilla, with oral implant and oral technique and extraction of tooth 25. The two central incisors were provisionally reconstructed with resin composite by the orthodontist.

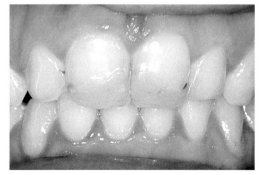

Fig 7-116   Vestibular view before restorative treatment.

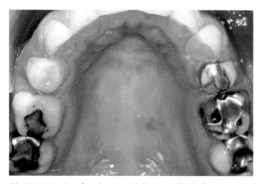

Fig 7-117 Occlusal view of the maxilla before restorative treatment.

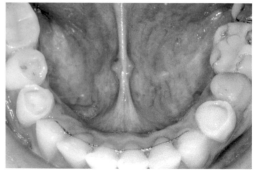

Fig 7-118 Occlusal view of the mandible before restorative treatment.

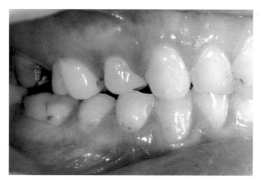

Fig 7-119 Right lateral view before restorative treatment.

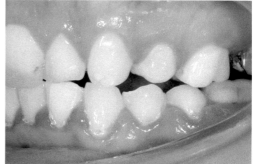

Fig 7-120 Left lateral view before restorative treatment.

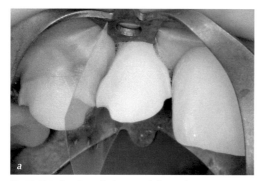

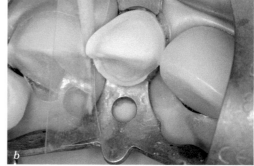

Fig 7-121a,b Detailed view while applying veneer crown to tooth 12.

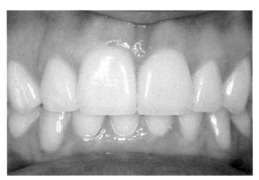

Fig 7-122 Vestibular view after restoration with veneer crowns in teeth 13 to 23.

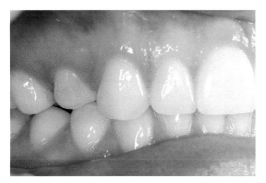

Fig 7-123 Right lateral view after restoration.

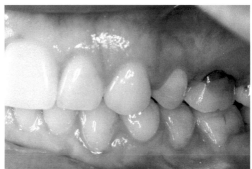

Fig 7-124 Left lateral view after restoration.

Case report 9
(Fig 7-125 to 7-139)

Composite overlays, direct resin composite reconstructions, and ceramic crowns

Carola Imfeld, Preventive Dentistry and Oral Epidemiology, University of Zurich

Diagnosis: multiple dental erosions on oral, occlusal, and vestibular tooth surfaces, partly combined with attrition.
Restorations: increase in vertical dimension by >2 mm, with the use of resin composite overlays and direct resin composite reconstructions; treatment of maxillary anterior teeth with full ceramic crowns.

Description

A 27-year-old woman with impaired dentition caused by an eating disorder required restoration of her dentition. The patient had been successfully treated by a psychiatrist and had been stable for some time. She continued psychotherapy, including a small daily dose of antidepressant. A dietary questionnaire also revealed other factors during the active phase of the disorder, such as the regular consumption of lemon juice with meals as well as large amounts of acidic fruits. At some stage, the patient had regularly performed mechanical oral hygiene immediately after acidic exposure. Additionally, a reflux condition had appeared intermittently as a result of the disorder. Bruxism was reported to have occurred in the past.

There was no indication of decreased salivary flow rate. A retainer in the mandibular anterior teeth was loose. Periodontal examination showed localized gingivitis and severe recessions in the anterior mandibular teeth. Maxillary as well as mandibular anterior teeth showed attrition as well as erosion.

Diagnosis

Advanced stage of intrinsic and extrinsic dental erosions, partially combined with abrasion; attrition in maxillary and mandibular anterior teeth; status after orthodontic therapy.

Therapy

During prior orthodontic examination, it was decided to remove the retainer and to strip the mandibular anterior teeth to enable retrusion, which would relieve the stress on the maxillary anterior teeth. After detailed information, the patient opted for minimally invasive treatment with resin composite reconstructions and overlays in all lateral teeth and the mandibular anterior teeth. The patient wanted full ceramic crowns in the maxillary anterior teeth despite the acknowledged high invasiveness of this treatment option. All adhesive restorations were performed using rubber-dam and total bonding. The treatment was performed as follows:

1. Direct resin composite fillings in hypersensitive cervical surfaces of teeth 33 to 37
2. Replacement of amalgam fillings in the maxilla by resin composite,

while simultaneously reconstruct-ing occlusal surfaces and vertical dimension

3. Treatment of cervical defect of tooth 26 orally with direct resin composite restoration

4. Replacement of amalgam fillings in teeth 37, 36, 46, and 47 by resin composite overlays, while simulta-neously reconstructing occlusal surfaces and vertical dimension

5. Direct resin composite reconstruc-tion of teeth 35 to 45 occlusally and incisally, while simultaneously replacing amalgam fillings in teeth 35 and 45

6. Full ceramic crowns for teeth 13 to 23

7. Provision of a Michigan splint for the maxilla to treat recurring bruxism.

Two and a half years after this therapy, the patient suffered a relapse of her eat-ing disorder and severe erosive expo-sure led to erosive defects primarily in the mandibular lateral teeth occlusally and buccally. Both the restorations and the dental hard tissue were affected. After stabilization of the condition, the defects were repaired with direct resin composite. Other measures and main-tenance were not necessary.

The patient presents three times per year for dental hygiene treatment and motivation as well as dietary coun-seling. Because of increasing dentin wear at the sites of gingival recession on the mandibular anterior teeth, a root coverage procedure is planned.

Discussion

The patient suffered from dental hard tissue loss through erosion, with con-tributions also from abrasion and attri-tion. Dental treatment was initiated once it was confirmed that the eating disorder had been stabilized. Only pro-phylactic measures are recommended during active eating disorders. A re-lapse caused damage in restorations as well as teeth. While ceramic recon-structions might have proved more du-rable (but not their surrounding tooth substance), they are more difficult to repair and require much more invasive preparatory measures. Additionally, bruxism can cause fractures in ceramic reconstructions. The reconstruction of the maxillary anterior teeth with full ceramic crowns is considered an inva-sive treatment. It was done here to meet the patient's wishes.

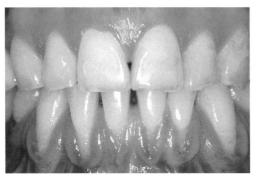

Fig 7-125 *Initial frontal view with vestibular erosions in maxillary teeth and gingiva recession in mandible.*

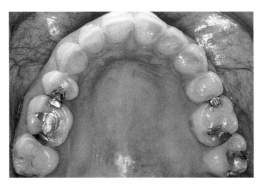

Fig 7-126 *Initial view of the maxilla, with generalized erosions and localized attrition in anterior teeth.*

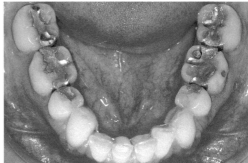

Fig 7-127 *Initial view of the mandible, with generalized erosions and localized attrition in anterior teeth.*

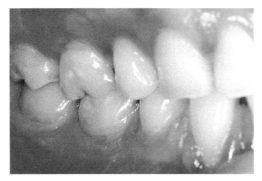

Fig 7-128 *Initial right lateral view with erosions.*

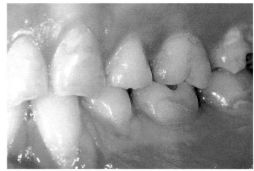

Fig 7-129 *Initial left lateral view with erosions.*

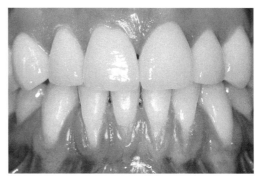

Fig 7-130 *Frontal view with full ceramic crowns in teeth 13 to 23 and direct resin composite filling buccally in tooth 33.*

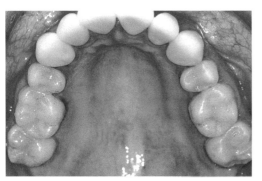

Fig 7-131 *Maxilla after direct resin composite reconstructions of lateral teeth.*

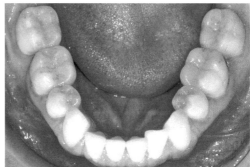

Fig 7-132 *Mandible after treatment of teeth 37, 36, 46, and 47 with resin composite overlays and direct resin composite reconstructions in teeth 35 to 45.*

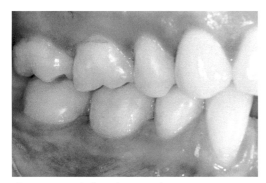

Fig 7-133 *Right lateral view with resin composite overlays in teeth 46 and 47 as well as direct resin composite reconstructions in remaining lateral teeth.*

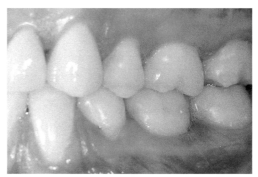

Fig 7-134 *Left lateral view with resin composite overlays in teeth 36 and 37 and direct resin composite reconstructions in remaining lateral teeth. Teeth 37 to 33 included resin composite fillings buccally.*

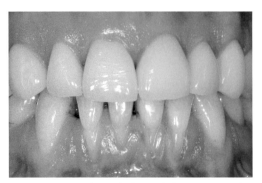

Fig 7-135 *Frontal view before polishing, 7 years after reconstruction.*

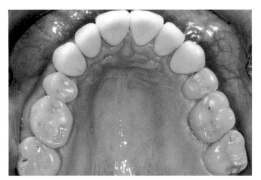

Fig 7-136 *Maxilla before polishing, 7 years after reconstruction.*

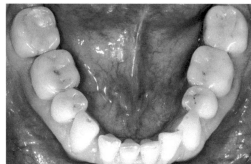

Fig 7-137 *Mandible before polishing, 7 years after reconstruction.*

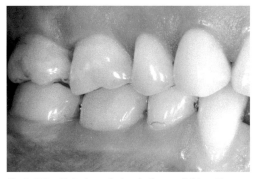

Fig 7-138 *Right lateral view before polishing, 7 years after reconstruction.*

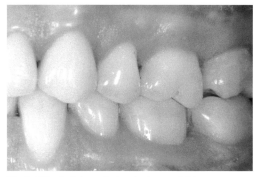

Fig 7-139 *Left lateral view before polishing, 7 years after reconstruction.*

References

1. Bartlett D, Ganß C, Lussi A. Basic erosive wear examination (BEWE): a new scoring system for scientific and clinical needs. Clin Oral Invest 2008;12:S65-S68.

2. Lussi A, Jaeggi T, Zero D. The role of diet in the aetiology of dental erosion. Caries Res 2004;38(Suppl 1):34–44.

3. Attin T, Buchalla W, Gollner M, Hellwig E. Use of variable remineralization periods to improve the abrasion resistance of previously eroded enamel. Caries Res 2000;34:48–52.

4. Davis WB, Winter PJ. The effect of abrasion on enamel and dentine and exposure to dietary acid. Br Dent J 1980;148:253–256.

5. Jaeggi T, Lussi A. Toothbrush abrasion of erosively altered enamel after intraoral exposure to saliva: an in situ study. Caries Res 1999;33:455–461.

6. Dugmore CR, Rock WP. The progression of tooth erosion in a cohort of adolescents of mixed ethnicity. Int J Paediatr Dent 2003;13:295–303.

7. El Aidi H, Bronkhorst EM, Truin GJ. A longitudinal study of tooth erosion in adolescents. J Dent Res 2008;87:731–735.

8. Ganß C, Klimek J, Giese K. Dental erosion in children and adolescents: a cross-sectional and longitudinal investigation using study models. Community Dent Oral Epidemiol 2001;29: 264–271.

9. Lussi A, Schaffner M. Progression of and risk factors for dental erosion and wedge-shaped defects over a 6-year period. Caries Res 2000;34: 182–187.

10. Nunn JH, Rugg-Gunn A, Gordon PH, Stephenson G. A longitudinal study of dental erosion in adolescent girls. Caries Res 2001;35:296 (ORCA Abstract 97).

11. Al-Dlaigan YH, Shaw L, Smith A. Dental erosion in a group of British 14-year-old, school children. Part I: prevalence and influence of differing socioeconomic backgrounds. Br Dent J 2001;190:145–149.

12. Arnadottir IB, Saemundsson SR, Holbrook WP. Dental erosion in Icelandic teenagers in relation to dietary and lifestyle factors. Acta Odontol Scand 2003;61:25–28.

13. Auad SM, Waterhouse PJ, Nunn JH, Stehen N, Moynihan PJ. Dental erosion amongst 13- and 14-year-old Brazilian schoolchildren. Int Dent J 2007;57:161–167.

14. Caglar E, Kargul B, Tanboga I, Lussi A. Dental erosion among children in an Istanbul public school. J Dent Child 2005;72:5–9.

15. Jaeggi T, Lussi A. Erosionen bei Kindern im frühen Schulalter. Schweiz Monatsschr Zahnmed 2004;114:876–881.

16. Jaeggi T, Schaffner M, Bürgin W, Lussi A. Erosionen und keilförmige Defekte bei Rekruten der Schweizer Armee. Schweiz Monatsschr Zahnmed 1999;109:1171–1182.

17. Larsen MJ, Poulsen S, Hansen I. Erosion of the teeth: prevalence and distribution in a group of Danish school children. Eur J Paediatr Dent 2005;6:44–47.

18. Lussi A, Schaffner M, Hotz P, Suter P. Dental erosion in a population of Swiss adults. Community Dent Oral Epidemiol 1991;19:286–290.

19. Millward A, Shaw L, Smith A. Dental erosion in four-year-old children from differing socioeconomic backgrounds. ASDC J Dent Child 1994;61:263–266.

20. Milosevic A, Young PJ, Lennon MA. The prevalence of tooth wear in 14-year-old school children in Liverpool. Community Dent Health 1994;11:83–86.

21. Nunn JH, Gordon PH, Morris AJ, Pine CM, Walker A. Dental erosion: changing prevalence? A review of British national childrens' surveys. Int J Paediatr Dent 2003;13:98–105.

22. Schiffner U, Micheelis W, Reich E. Erosionen und keilförmige Zahnhalsdefekte bei deutschen Erwachsenen und Senioren. Dtsch Zahnärztl Z 2002;57:102–106.

23. van Rijkom HM, Truin GJ, Frencken JEFM, et al. Prevalence, distribution and background variables of smooth-bordered tooth wear in teenagers in The Hague, the Netherlands. Caries Res 2002;36:147–154.

24. Wiegand A, Müller J, Werner C, Attin T. Prevalence of erosive tooth wear and associated risk factors in 2–7-year-old German kindergarten children. Oral Diseases 2006;12:117–124.

25. Xhonga FA, Valdmanis S. Geographic comparisons of the incidence of dental erosion: a two centre study. J Oral Rehabil 1983;10:269–277.

26. Al-Malik MI, Holt RD, Bedi R. Erosion, caries and rampant caries in preschool children in Jeddah, Saudi Arabia. Community Dent Oral Epidmiol 2002;30:16–23.

27. Bardsley PF, Taylor S, Milosevic A. Epidemiological studies of tooth wear and dental erosion in 14-year-old children in North West England. Part 1: the relationship with water fluoridation and social deprivation. Br Dent J 2004;197: 413–416.

28. Chadwick RG, Mitchell HL, Manton SL, Ward S, Ogston S, Brown R. Maxillary incisor palatal erosion: no correlation with dietary variables? J Clin Pediatr Dent 2005;29:157–164.

29. Deery C, Wagner ML, Longbottom C, Simon R, Nugent ZJ. The prevalence of dental erosion in a United States and a United Kingdom sample of adolescents. Pediatr Dent 2000;22: 505–510.

30. Dugmore CR, Rock WP. The prevalence of tooth erosion in 12-year-old children. Br Dent J 2004;196:279–282.

31. El Karim IA, Sanhouri NM, Hashim NT, Ziada HM. Dental erosion among 12–14 year old school children in Khartoum: a pilot study. Community Dent Health 2007;24:176–180.

32. Harding MA, Whelton H, O'Mullane DM, Cronin M. Dental erosion in 5-year-old Irish school children and associated factors: a pilot study. Community Dent Health 2003;20:165–170.

33. Johansson AK, Johansson A, Birkhed D, Omar R, Baghdadi S, Carlsson GE. Dental erosion, soft drink intake, and oral health in young Saudi men, and the development of a system for assessing erosive anterior tooth wear. Acta Odontol Scand 1996;54:369–378.

34. Kazoullis S, Seow WK, Holcombe T, Newman B, Ford D. Common dental conditions associated with dental erosion in schoolchildren in Australia. Pediatr Dent 2007;29:33–39.

35. Luo Y, Zeng XJ, Du MQ, Bedi R. The prevalence of dental erosion in preschool children in China. J Dent 2005;33:115–121.

36. Truin GJ, Frencken JE, Mulder J, Kootwijk AJ, Jong E. Prevalence of caries and dental erosion among school children in The Hague from 1996 to 2005. Ned Tijdschr Tandheelkd 2007;114: 335–342.

37. Truin GJ, van Rijkom HM, Mulder J, van't Hof MA. Caries trends 1996–2002 among 6- and 12-year-old children and erosive wear prevalence among 12-year-old children in The Hague. Caries Res 2005;39:2–8.

38. Williams D, Croucher R, Marcenes W, O'Farrell M. The prevalence of dental erosion in the maxillary incisors of 14-year-old schoolchildren living in Tower Hamlets and Hackney, London, UK. Int Dent J 1999;49:211–216.

39. Xhonga FA, Wolcott RB, Sognnaes RF. Dental erosion. II. Clinical measurements of dental erosion progress. J Am Dent Assoc 1972;84:577–582.

40. Dugmore CR, Rock WP. A multifactorial analysis of factors associated with dental erosion. Br Dent J 2004;196:283–286.

41. Ganß C, Schlechtriemen M, Klimek J. Dental erosions in subjects living on a raw food diet. Caries Res 1999;33:74–80.

42. Edwards M, Ashwood RA, Littlewood SJ, Brocklebank LM, Fung DE. A videofluoroscopic comparison of straw and cup drinking: the potential influence on dental erosion. Br Dent J 1998;185: 244–249.

43. Johansson AK, Lingström P, Imfeld T, Birkhed D. Influence of drinking method on tooth-surface pH in relation to dental erosion. Eur J Oral Sci 2004;112:484–489.

44. Millward A, Shaw L, Harrington E, Smith AJ. Continuous monitoring of salivary flow rate and pH at the surface of the dentition following consumption of acidic beverages. Caries Res 1997;31:44–49.

45. Vakil N, van Zanten SV, Kahrilas P, Dent J, Jones R for the Global Consensus Group. The Montreal definition and classification of gastroesophageal reflux disease: a global evidence-based consensus. Am J Gastroenterol 2006; 101:1900–1920.

46. Rai AM, Orlando RC. Gastroesophageal reflux disease. Curr Opin Gastroenterol 2001;17: 359–365.

47. Storr M, Meinung A, Allescher HD. Pharmacoeconomic issues of the treatment of gastroesophageal reflux disease. Expert Opin Pharmacother 2001;2:1099–1108.

48. Tsou VM, Bishop PR. Gastroesophageal reflux in children. Otolaryngol Clin North Am 1998;31:419–434.

49. Osatakul S, Sriplung H, Puetpaiboon A, Junjana CO, Chamnongpakdi S. Prevalence and natural

course of gastroesophageal reflux symptoms: a 1-year cohort study in Thai infants. J Pediatr Gastroenterol Nutr 2002;34:63–67.

50. Buttar NS, Falk GW. Pathogenesis of gastroesophageal reflux and Barrett esophagus. Mayo Clin Proc 2001;76:226–234.

51. Huang JQ, Hunt RH. pH, healing rate, and symptom relief in patients with GERD. Yale J Biol Med 1999;72:181–194.

52. Szarka LA, De Vault KR, Murray JA. Diagnosing gastroesophageal reflux disease. Mayo Clin Proc 2001;76:97–101.

53. Vandenplas Y. Oesophageal pH monitoring for gastro-oesophageal reflux in infants and children. Chichester, UK: Wiley, 1992.

54. Bartlett DW, Evans DF, Anggiansah A, Smith BG. A study of the association between gastro-oesophageal reflux and palatal dental erosion. Br Dent J 1996;181:125–131.

55. Katz PO. Lessons learned from intragastric pH monitoring. J Clin Gastroenterol 2001;33: 107- 113.

56. Schindlbeck NE. Optimal thresholds, sensitivity, and specificity of longterm pH-metry for the detection of gastroesophageal reflux disease. Gastroenterology 1987;93:85–90.

57. Cooper PJ, Charnock J, Taylor MJ. The prevalence of bulimia nervosa. Br J Psychiatry 1987;151:684–686.

58. Hellström I. Oral complications in anorexia nervosa. Scand J Dent Res 1977;8:71–86.

59. Jones RR, Cleaton-Jones P. Depth and areas of dental erosions and dental caries in bulimic women. J Dent Res 1989;68:1275–1278.

60. Milosevic A, Slade PD. The orodental status of anorexis and bulimics. Br Dent J 1989;67:66–70.

61. Robb N, Smith BGN, Geidrys-Leeper E. The distribution of erosion in the dentitons of patients with eating disorders. Br Dent J 1995;178: 171–175.

62. Scheutzel P. Zahnmedizinische Befunde bei psychogenen Essstörungen. Dtsch Zahnärztl Z 1992;47:119–123.

63. Abrams RA, Ruff JC. Oral signs and symtoms in the diagnosis of bulimia. J Am Dent Assoc 1986;113:761–764.

64. Lee M, Feldman M. Nausea and vomiting. In: Feldman M, Scharschmidt B, Sleisenger M (eds). Sleisenger and Fordstran's Gastrointestinal and Liver Disease: Pathophysiology, Diagnosis, Management, 6th edn. Philadelphia, PA: Saunders, 1998:117–127.

65. Eisenburger M, Addy M, Hughes JA, Shellis RP. Effect of time on the remineralisation of enamel by synthetic saliva after citric acid erosion. Caries Res 2001;35:211–215.

66. Feagin F, Koulourides T, Pigman W. The characterization of enamel surface demineralization, remineralization, and associated hardness changes in human and bovine material. Arch Oral Biol 1969;14:1407–1417.

67. Gedalia I, Dakuar A, Shapira L, Lewinsten I, Goultshin J, Rahamim E. Enamel softening with Coca-Cola and rehardening with milk or saliva. Am J Dent 1991;4:120–122.

68. Järvinen VK, Rytömaa II, Heinonen OP. Risk factors in dental erosion. J Dent Res 1991;70: 942–947.

69. Meurman J, Toskala J, Nuutinen P, Klemetti E. Oral and dental manifestations in gastroesophageal reflux disease. Oral Surg Oral Med Oral Pathol 1994;78:583–589.

70. Zero DT, Fu J, Scott-Anne K, Proskin H. Evaluation of fluoride dentifrices using a short-term intraoral remineralization model. J Dent Res 1994;73(Special issue):272.

71. Zero DT, Lussi A. Etiology of enamel erosion: intrinsic and extrinsic factors. In: Addy M, Embery G, Edgar WM, Orchardson R (eds). Tooth Wear and Sensitivity. London: Martin Dunitz, 2000:121–139.

72. Amaechi BT, Higham SM, Edgar WM, Milosevic A. Thickness of acquired salivary pellicle as a determinant of the sites of dental erosion. J Dent Res 1999;78:1821–1828.

73. Voronets J, Jaeggi T, Buergin W, Lussi A. Controlled toothbrush abrasion of softened human enamel. Caries Res 2008;42:286–290.

74. Westergaard J, Larsen IB, Holmen L, et al. Occupational exposure to airborne proteolytic enzymes and lifestyle risk factors for dental erosion: a cross-sectional study. Occup Med 2001;51:189–197.

75. Wiegand A, Begic M, Attin T. In vitro evaluation of abrasion of eroded ernamel by different manual, power and sonic toothbrushes. Caries Res 2006;40:60–65.

76. Union of European Soft Drinks Associations. www.unesda.org.

77. Meurman JH, ten Cate JM. Pathogenesis and modifying factors of dental erosion. Eur J Oral Sci 1996;104:199–206.

78. Lussi A, Jaeggi T, Jaeggi-Schärer S. Prediction of the erosive potential of some beverages. Caries Res 1995;29:349–354.

79. Lussi A, Jaeggi T, Schärer S. The influence of different factors on in vitro enamel erosion. Caries Res 1993;27:387–393.

80. Mahoney E, Beattie J, Swain M, Kilpatrick N. Preliminary in vitro assessment of erosive potential using the ultra-micro-indentation system. Caries Res 2003;37:218–224.

123

81. Hooper SM, West NX, Sharif N et al. A comparison of enamel erosion by a new sports drink compared to two proprietary products: a controlled, crossover study in situ. J Dent 2004;32:541–545.

82. Ramalingam L, Messer LB, Reynolds EC. Adding casein phosphopeptide–amorphous calcium phosphate to sports drinks to eliminate in vitro erosion. Pediatr Dent 2005;27:61–67.

83. Venables MC, Shaw L, Jeukendrup AE, et al. Erosive effect of a new sports drink on dental enamel during exercise. Med Sci Sports Exerc 2005;37:39–44.

84. Parry J, Shaw L, Arnaud MJ, Smith AJ. Investigation of mineral waters and soft drinks in relation to dental erosion. J Oral Rehabil 2001;28:766–772.

85. Lussi A, Megert B, Shellis RP, Wang X. Analysis of the erosive effect of different dietary substances and medications. Br J Nutr 2011 Jun 30 [Epub ahead of print].

86. Arowojolu MO. Erosion of tooth enamel surfaces among battery chargers and automobile mechanics in Ibadan: a comparative study. Afr J Med Med Sci 2001;30:5–8.

87. Amin WM, Al-Omoush SA, Hattab FN. Oral health status of workers exposed to acid fumes in phosphate and battery industries in Jordan. Int Dent J 2001;51:169–174.

88. Tuominen M, Tuominen R, Fubusa F, Mgalula N. Tooth surface loss exposure to organic and inorganic acid fumes in workplace air. Community Dent Oral Epidemiol 1991;19:217–220.

89. Tuominen M, Tuominen R, Ranta K, Ranta H. Association between acid fumes in the work environment and dental erosion. Scand J Work Environ Health 1989;15:335–338.

90. Tuominen M, Tuominen R. Dental erosion and associated factors among factory workers exposed to inorganic acid fumes. Proc Finn Dent Soc 1991;87:359–364.

91. Petersen PE, Gormsen C. Oral conditions among German battery factory workers. Community Dent Oral Epidemiol 1991;19:104–106.

92. Wiegand A, Attin T. Occupational dental erosion from exposure to acids: a review. Occup Med 2007;57:169–176.

93. Wiktorsson AM, Zimmerman M, Angmar-Mansson B. Erosive tooth wear: prevalence and severity in Swedish winetasters. Eur J Oral Sci 1997;105:544–550.

94. Chaudhry SI, Harris JL, Challacombe SJ. Dental erosion in a wine merchant: an occupational hazard? Br Dent J 1997;182:226–228.

95. Ferguson MM, Dunbar RJ, Smith JA, Wall JG. Enamel erosion related to winemaking. Occup Med 1996;46:159–162.

96. Gray A, Ferguson MM, Wall JG. Wine tasting and dental erosion. Case Report. Aust Dent J 1998;43:32–34.

97. Coombes JS, Hamilton KL. The effectiveness of commercially available sports drinks. Sports Med 2000;29:181–209.

98. Coombes JS. Sports drinks and dental erosion. Am J Dent 2005;18:101–104.

99. Pugh LG, Corbett JL, Johnson RH. Rectal temperatures, weight losses, and sweat rates in marathon running. J Appl Physiol 1967;23:347–352.

100. Sirimaharaj V, Brearley Messer L, Morgan MV. Acidic diet and dental erosion among athletes. Aust Dent J 2002;47:228–236.

101. Milosevic A, Kelly MJ, McLean AN. Sports supplement drinks and dental health in competitive swimmers and cyclists. Br Dent J 1997;182: 303–308.

102. Mathew T, Casamassimo PS, Hayes JR. Relationship between sports drinks and dental erosion in 304 university athletes in Columbus, Ohio, USA. Caries Res 2002;36:281–287.

103. Hooper SM, Hughes JA, Newcombe RG, Addy M, West NX. A methodology for testing the erosive potential of sports drinks. J Dent 2005;33: 343–348.

104. Geurtsen W. Rapid general dental erosion by gas-chlorinated swimming pool water. Review of the literature and case report. Am J Dent 2000;13:291–293.

105. Centerwall BS, Armstrong CW, Funkhouser LS, Elzay RP. Erosion of dental enamel among competitive swimmers at a gas-chlorinated swimming pool. Am J Epidemiol 1986;123:641–647.

106. Deibert P, König D, Allgaier HP, Berg A. Sport and the digestive system. Dtsch Med Wochenschr 2007;132:155–160.

107. Clark CS, Kraus BB, Sinclair J, Castell DO. Gastroesophageal reflux induced by exercise in healthy volunteers. JAMA 1989;261:3599–3601.

108. Lutz F, Krejci I. Resin composites in the postamalgam age. Compend Contin Educ Dent 1999;20:1138–1148.

109. O'Sullivan EA, Curzon MEJ. A comparison of acidic dietary factors in children with and without dental erosion. J Dent Child 2000;67:186–192.

110. Barbour ME, Finke M, Parker DM, Hughes JA, Allen GC, Addy M. The relationship between enamel softening and erosion caused by soft drinks at a range of temperatures. J Dent 2006;34: 207–213.

111. Amaechi BT, Higham SM, Edgar WM. The influence of xylitol and fluoride on dental erosion in vitro. Arch Oral 1998;43:157–161.

112. Bartlett DW, Evans DF, Smith BG. The relationship between gastro-oesphageal reflux disease and dental erosion. J Oral Rehabil 1996;23: 289–297.

113. DeMeester TR. Technique, indications and clinical use of 24 hour esophageal pH monitoring. J Thorac Cardiovasc Surg 1980;79:656–670.

114. Faubion WA, Zein NN. Gastroesophageal reflux in infants and children. Mayo Clin Proc 1998;73: 66–173.

115. Röhss K, Wilder-Smith C, Claar-Nilsson C, Hasselgren G. Esomeprazole 40 mg provides more effective acid control than standard doses of all other proton pump inhibitors. Gastroenterology 2001;120:A419.

116. Bell NJV, Burget D, Howden CW, Wilkinson J, Hunt RH. Appropriate acid suppression for the management of gastrooesophageal reflux disease. Digestion 1992;51:59–67.

117. Lussi A, Megert B, Eggenberger D, Jaeggi T. Impact of different toothpaste on the prevention of erosion. Caries Res 2008;42:62–67.

118. Wiegand A, Egert S, Attin T. Toothbrushing before or after an acidic challenge to minimize tooth wear? An in situ/ex vivo study. Am J Dent 2008;21:13–16.

119. Joiner J, Schwaz A, Philpotts CJ, Cox TF, Huber K, Hannig M. The protective nature of pellicle towards toothpaste abrasion on enamel and dentine. J Dent 2008;36:360–368.

120. Ganß C, Klimek J, Schäffer U, Spall T. Effectiveness of two fluoridation measures on erosion progression in human enamel and dentine in vitro. Caries Res 2001;35:325–330.

121. Petzold M. The influence of different fluoride compounds and treatment conditions on dental enamel: a descriptive in vitro study of the CaF_2 precipitation and microstructure. Caries Res 2001;35:45–51.

122. Lussi A, Hellwig E. Erosive potential of oral care products. Caries Res 2001;35(Suppl 1):52–56.

123. Ganß C, Schlueter N, Hardt M, Schattenberg P, Klimek J. Effect of fluoride compounds on enamel erosion in vitro: a comparison of amine, sodium and stannous fluoride. Caries Res 2008; 42:2–7.

124. Schlueter N, Duran A, Klimek J, Ganß C. Investigation of the effect of various fluoride compounds and preparations thereof on erosive tissue loss in enamel in vitro. Caries Res 2009;43:10–16.

125. Neuhaus KW, Lussi A. Casein Phosphopeptid–Amorphes Calcium phosphat (CPP-ACP) und seine Wirkung auf die Zahnhartsubstanz. Schweiz Monatsschr Zahnmed 2009;119.

126. Moazzez R, Bartlett D, Anggiansah A. The effect of chewing sugar-free gum on gastro-esophageal reflux. J Dent Res 2005;84:1062–1065.

127. Jensdottir T, Nauntofte B, Buchwald C, Hansen HS, Bardow A. Effects of sucking acidic candies on saliva in unilaterally irradiated pharyngeal cancer patients. Oral Oncol 2006;42:317–322.

128. Lussi A, Portmann P, Burhop B. Erosion on abraded dental hard tissues by acid lozenges: an in situ study. Clin Oral Invest 1997;1:191–194.

129. Sundaram G, Wilson R, Watson TF, Bartlett D. Clinical measurement of palatal tooth wear following coating by a resin sealing system. Oper Dent 2007;32:539–543.

130. Amaechi BT, Higham SM, Edgar WM. Factors influencing the development of dental erosion in vitro: enamel type, temperature and exposure time. J Oral Rehabil 1999;26:624–630.

131. Hunter ML, West NX, Hughes JA, Newcombe RG, Addy M. Erosion of deciduous and permanent dental hard tissue in the oral environment. J Dent 2000;28:257–263.

132. Hunter ML, West NX, Hughes JA, Newcombe RG, Addy M. Relative susceptibility of deciduous and permanent dental hard tissues to erosion by a low pH fruit drink in vitro. J Dent 2000;28: 265–270.

133. Lussi A, Kohler N, Zero D, Schaffner M, Megert B. A comparison of the erosive potential of different beverages in primary and permanent teeth using an in vitro model. Eur J Oral Sci 2000;108: 110–114.

134. Dahshan A, Patel H, Delaney J, Wuerth A, Thomas R, Tolia V. Gastroesophageal reflux disease and dental erosion in children. J Pediatr 2002;140:474–478.

135. Ersin NK, Onçag O, Tügmgör G, Aydogdu S, Hilmioglu S. Oral and dental manifestations of gastroesophageal reflux disease in children: a preliminary study. Pediatr Dent 2006;28:279–284.

136. Linnett V, Seow WK. Dental erosion in children: a literature review. Pediatr Dent 2001;23: 37–43.

137. Tay FR, Pashley DH. Resin bonding to cervical sclerotic dentin: a review. J Dent 2004;32: 173–196.

138. Ogata M, Okuda M, Nakajima M, Pereira PN, Sano H, Tagami J. Influence of the direction of tubules on bond strength to dentin. Oper Dent 2001;26:27–35.

139. Ogata M, Harada N, Yamaguchi S, Nakajima M, Pereira PN, Tagami J. Effects of different burs on dentin bond strengths of self-etching primer bonding systems. Oper Dent 2001;26:375–382.

140. Soderholm KJ, Richards ND. Wear resistance of composites: a solved problem? Gen Dent 1998;46:256–263.

141. Gaengler P, Hoyer I, Montag R. Clinical evaluation of posterior composite restorations: the 10-year report. J Adhes Dent 2001;3:185–194.

142. Matis BA, Cochran M, Carlson T. Longevity of glass-ionomer restorative materials: results of a 10-year evaluation. Quintessence Int 1996;27:373–382.

143. Opdam NJK, Bronkhorst EM, Roeters JM, Loomans BAC. A retrospective clinical study on longevity of posterior composite and amalgam restorations. Dent Mat 2007;23:2–8.

144. Fasbinder DJ. Clinical performance of chairside CAD/CAM restorations. J Am Dent Assoc 2006;137:22S–31S.

145. Manhart J, Chen H, Hamm G, Hickel R. Buonocore Memorial Lecture. Review of the clinical survival of direct and indirect restorations in posterior teeth of the permanent dentition. Oper Dent 2004;29:481–508.

146. Mjör IA, Davis MR, Abu-Hanna A. CAD/CAM restorations and secondary caries: a literature review with illustrations. Dent Update 2008;35:118–120.

147. Manhart J, Hickel R. Longevity of restorations. In: Roulet JF, Wilson NHF, Fuzzi M (eds). Advances in Operative Dentistry 2001, Vol. 2: Challenges of the Future. Chicago, IL: Quintessence, 2001;45–64.

148. Nomoto R, McCabe JF. A simple acid erosion test for dental water-based cements. Dent Mat 2001;17:53–59.

149. Al-Hiyasat AS, Saunders WP, Sharkey SW, Smith GM. The effect of a carbonated beverage on the wear of human enamel and dental ceramics. J Prosthodont 1998;7:2–12.

150. Shabanian M, Richards LC. In vitro wear rates of materials under different loads and varying pH. J Prosthet Dent 2002;87:650–656.

151. Yap AU, Tan SHL, Wee SSC, Lee CW, Lim ELC, Zeng KY. Chemical degradation of composite restoratives. J Oral Rehabil 2001;28:1015–1021.

152. Aliping-McKenzie M, Linden RWA, Nicholson JW. The effect of Coca-Cola and fruit juices on the surface hardness of glass-ionomers and "compomers." J Oral Rehabil 2004;31:1046–1052.

153. Gomec Y, Dorter C, Ersev H, Guray Efes B, Yildiz E. Effects of dietary acids on surface microhardness of various tooth-colored restoratives. Dent Mater J 2004; 23:429–435.

154. Mohamed-Tahir MA, Tan HY, Woo AA, Yap AU. Effects of pH on the microhardness of resin-based restorative materials. Oper Dent 2005;30: 661–666.

155. Wongkhantee S, Patanapiradej V, Maneenut C, Tantbirojn D. Effect of acidic food and drinks on surface hardness of enamel, dentine, and tooth coloured filling materials. J Dentistry 2006;34:214–220.

156. Francisconi LF, Honório HM, Rios D, Magalhães AC, Machado MA, Buzalaf MA. Effect of erosive pH cycling on different restorative materials and on enamel restored with these materials. Oper Dent 2008;33:203–208.

157. Rios D, Honorio HM, Francisconi LF, Magalhaes AC, De Andrade Moreira Machado MA, Buzalaf MAR. In situ effect of an erosive challenge on different restorative materials and on enamel adjacent to these materials. J Dent 2008;36:152–157.

158. Turssi CP, Hara AT, Serra MC, Rodrigues AL Jr. Effect of storage media upon the surface micromorphology of resin-based restorative materials. J Oral Rehabil 2002;29:864–871.

159. Mohamed-Tahir MA, Yap AU. Effects of pH on the surface texture of glass ionomer based/containing restorative materials. Oper Dent 2004;29:586–591.

160. Prakki A, Cilli R, de Araujo PA, Navarro MF, Mondelli J, Mondelli RF. Effect of toothbrushing abrasion on weight and surface roughness of pH cycled resin cements and indirect restorative materials. Quintessence Int 2007;38:544–554.

161. Lambrechts P, Van Meerbeek B, Perdigao J, Gladys S, Braem M, Vanherle G. Restorative therapy for erosive lesions. Eur J Oral Sci 1996;104:229–240.

162. Yip KH, Smales RJ, Kaidonis JA. The diagnosis and control of extrinsic acid erosion of tooth substance. Quintessence Int 2002;33:516–520.

163. Dahl BL, Krogstad O. The effect of partial bite raising splint on the occlusal face height. An X-ray cephalometric study in human adults. Acta Odontol Scand 1982;40:17–24.

164. Bartlett DW. The role of erosion in tooth wear: aetiology, prevention and management. Int Dent J 2005;4:277–284.

165. Ganddini MR, Al-Mardini M, Graser GN, Almong D. Maxillary and mandibular overlay removable partial dentures for the restoration of worn teeth. J Prost Dent 2004;91:210–214.

166. Hugo B. Orale Rehabilitation einer Erosionssituation. Schweiz Monatsschr Zahnmed 1991;101:1155–1162.

167. Kavoura V, Kourtis SG, Zoidis P, Andritsakis DP, Doukoudakis A. Full-mouth rehabilitation of a patient with bulimia nervosa. A case report. Quintessence Int. 2005;36:501–510.

168. Manhart J, Garcia-Godoy F, Hickel R. Direct posterior restorations: clinical results and new developments. Dent Clin North Am 2002;46:303–339.

169. Aziz K, Ziebert AJ, Cobb D. Restoring erosion associated with gastroesophageal reflux using direct resins: case report. Oper Dent 2005;30: 395–401.

170. Bartlett DW. Three patient reports illustrating the use of dentine adhesives to cement crowns to severely worn teeth. Int J Prosthodont 2005;18:214–218.

171. Hastings JH. Conservative restoration of function and aesthetics in a bulimic patient: a case report. Pract Periodontics Aesthet Dent 1996;8: 729–736.

172. Tepper SA, Schmidlin PR. Technik der direkten Bisshöhenrekonstruktion mit Komposit und einer Schiene als Formhilfe. Schweiz Monatsschr Zahnmed 2005;115:35–42.

173. Sundaram G, Wilson R, Watson TF, Bartlett D. Clinical measurement of palatal tooth wear following coating by a resin sealing system. Oper Dent 2007;32:539–543.

174. Yip HK, Lam WTC, Smales RJ. Fluoride release, weight loss and erosive wear of modern aesthetic restoratives. Br Dent J 1999;187:265–270.

175. Montgomery MT, Ritvo J, Weiner K. Eating disorders: phenomenology, identification, and dental intervention. Gen Dent 1988;36:485–488.

176. Schmidlin PR, Filli T. Direkte Bisshöhenrekonstruktion mit Komposit und Schiene als Formhilfe. Zahnärztl Mitteilungen 2006;96:30–34.

177. Schmidlin PR, Filli T, Imfeld C, Tepper S, Attin T. Three-year evaluation of posterior vertical bite reconstruction using direct resin composite: a case series. Oper Dent 2009;34:102–108.

178. Gavish A, Winocur E, Ventura YS, Halachmi M, Gazit E. Effect of stabilization splint therapy on pain during chewing in patients suffering from myofascial pain. J Oral Rehabil 2002;29:1181–1186.

179. Miller VJ. Treatment dentures: acrylic partial denture and stabilization splint. J Prosthet Dent 1992;67:736–737.

180. Hickel R, Manhart J. Longevity of restorations in posterior teeth and reasons for failure. J Adhes Dent 2001;3:45–64.

181. Brunthaler A, König F, Lucas T, Sperr W, Schedle A. Longevity of direct resin composite restorations in posterior teeth. Clin Oral Invest 2003;7:63–70.

182. Ganß C, Klimek J, Brune V, Schürmann A. Effects of two fluoridation measures on erosion progression in human enamel and dentine in situ. Caries Res 2004;38:561–566.

Index